OF MANY MINDS

Of Many Minds

NEURODIVERSITY AND MENTAL HEALTH AMONG
FACULTY AND STAFF

Edited by Rebecca Pope-Ruark
and Lee Skallerup Bessette
Foreword by Katie Rose Guest Pryal

JOHNS HOPKINS UNIVERSITY PRESS | *Baltimore*

© 2025 Johns Hopkins University Press
All rights reserved. Published 2025
Printed in the United States of America on acid-free paper
9 8 7 6 5 4 3 2 1

Johns Hopkins University Press
2715 North Charles Street
Baltimore, Maryland 21218
www.press.jhu.edu

Library of Congress Cataloging-in-Publication Data is available.

ISBN 978-1-4214-5252-4 (hardcover)
ISBN 978-1-4214-5253-1 (ebook)

A catalog record for this book is available from the British Library.

Special discounts are available for bulk purchases of this book.
For more information, please contact Special Sales at specialsales@jh.edu.

EU GPSR Authorized Representative
LOGOS EUROPE, 9 rue Nicolas Poussin, 17000, La Rochelle, France
E-mail: Contact@logoseurope.eu

CONTENTS

FOREWORD

KATIE ROSE GUEST PRYAL

As I write this foreword, I am starting my second week of antidepressants. I tell you this for two reasons. First, many of you will not know how hard it is to write when you are depressed. Sometimes, like today, it is difficult.

Sometimes, it is impossible.

The second reason I am telling you about depression and antidepressants is because of stigma. Stigma against neurodivergent people has so soaked into the fabric of our society that most people, including neurodivergent people, fail to even notice it. I define stigma against neurodivergent people as a process that creates negative stereotyping and isolation, typically based on the irrational fear of undesirable behavior such as irresponsibility, instability, or violence. Stigma also works internally on disabled people, creating feelings of isolation and shame (Pryal 2024a).

So by telling you that I am taking antidepressants and that I have depression now—even as I write the foreword to this fancy book being published by a highfalutin press—I am letting you know that it is entirely possible for someone whose brain is not firing on all cylinders to be quite capable of doing good things, even magnificent things. (Although I make no claims that this foreword will be magnificent.)

You will find in this book many magnificent things written by neurodivergent faculty and staff that will help you understand what neurodiversity is and how it affects higher education. Reading these stories will help break down the stigma against neurodiversity, both within the academy and without. We cannot ask more from this or any book.

* * *

I first publicly shared my own neurodiversity and started writing about it in 2014, which coincided with leaving my full-time contingent faculty position in higher education. I kept my bipolar disorder under wraps while working in both law and higher education because I was afraid. Like many neurodivergent faculty, I feared that my colleagues would think less of me; that I would be treated poorly by the administration; and that I would lose credibility in the classroom.

I define "neurodiversity" as normal variations in human neurological function, emphasis on *normal* (Pryal 2024c). Although the term, a portmanteau of "neurological diversity," first came into popularity in the context of autism, neurodiversity is a generous word that encompasses not only developmental neurodivergences, such as autism and attention deficit hyperactivity disorder, but also psychiatric ones, such as bipolar disorder and anxiety, and acquired ones such as post-traumatic stress disorder and brain fog.

Not all normal variations in human-ness are treated the same. Some variations are penalized. Neurodiversity is one of them. To have a brain that deviates from the socially constructed "normal" brain means that you are made wrong. You are then stigmatized, that is, punished for your differences. And in higher education, where we live by Descartes's *cogito, ergo sum*, if you cannot think properly, then you do not *exist* properly.

I never disclosed my neurodivergence at my higher education workplace for just this reason. I was afraid that I would be fired. To some of you, that fear might sound dramatic, but it is not. Sure, you would think that no one would be reckless enough to walk up to any employee and say, "We're letting you go because you have bipolar disorder." That is just asking for a lawsuit, especially in a law firm or a law school (where I taught). But that is not usually how job discrimination works.

If you have been subject to discrimination these days, then you know it is not about what people say out loud. It is about what people do not say, how they talk *around* what they mean. They would call me unreliable. "We can't count on you to complete this committee work," conjuring up some moment when I did not finish a project on time. It matters little that everyone gets behind sometimes, or that I rarely ever do. Just one strike against me would be enough. They would say to me, "You've been acting erratic lately and making your colleagues uncomfortable." Erratic. Uncomfortable. All these words compose the coded language used to alienate neurodivergent people. These are the words that employers use to make a case against us.

When they do fire you and you know it is because you are neurodivergent and have bipolar disorder, depression, anxiety, or autism, you cannot afford to sue, and they know that too. Employment lawsuits are expensive and emotionally taxing. Most of us would walk away. So we have to pick ourselves up and move on.

*   *   *

How do we avoid these risks caused by stigma against neurodivergent people? We hide, as best we can, the traits that make us who we are. We *mask*. Masking occurs when neurodivergent people hide their neurodivergent traits to appease neurotypical norms because they will face negative consequences if they do not—which is almost always.

As Dr. Lee Skallerup Bessette writes in the introduction to this book, in higher education "the masking is seemingly easier, at least at first, and fuels a neurotypical view of ourselves—if I can just do these things, I will be accepted in this space." But as she puts it, "Higher education is a trap for neurodivergent people" because in the end, although "academia at least makes gestures toward inclusivity . . . it is still a system steeped in ableism." Higher education just hides it better until it traps neurodivergent faculty in its web.

Dr. Catherine Denial writes in her chapter of this book that it is the neurodivergent faculty member's inescapable burden to mask: "I was working so hard every day to show up and teach all my classes; it was an unbearable struggle to write my lectures and get out of my front door." But she did not let her battle show: "I was masking—desperately presenting an appearance of mental health and/or neurotypicality to others so that I would be accepted and stay employed." As Denial explains, job security was always at the forefront. I can relate. We *all* can relate. But the problem is that no matter how hard we try, it is never good enough. Denial writes: "I was doing everything I could to be the right kind of professor while scared that it was an impossible task."

After I spent years masking, overworking to compensate for my fear of failing to be a good professor, I left to work for myself, which was terrifying but also freeing. I could finally be my complete self. In 2014

I wrote an article for the *Chronicle of Higher Education*, "Disclosure Blues," in which I shared that I had bipolar disorder (Pryal 2014). The response to the piece was immense: private messages on social media and emails to me, all from people who felt as I had—that they spend their days suffering because they fear for their jobs, living not only in perpetual anxiety but also perpetual exhaustion from hiding—masking—who they really are.

The *Chronicle* essay was published more than a decade ago, when the subject of neurodiversity was even more taboo than it is now. I interviewed multiple faculty members who had finally come out to their institutions with their neurodivergences and others who had not, and what we all concluded was this: Do not disclose unless you must in order to receive accommodations or unless you have bulletproof job security—that is, tenure. And even then, be careful because some of your colleagues *will* treat you differently. Ableism and stigma permeate the academy, and even tenure cannot protect you from those.

Because I define "faculty" as *any* person whose job it is to educate students, be they advisers, librarians, teachers, or administrative staff, the vast majority of neurodivergent faculty do not have the job security of tenure.

Even when I finally had the freedom to write about my bipolar disorder because I knew I could not be fired for it, I was still terrified. If you had asked me then what I was afraid of, I would not have been able to tell you. But looking back now, I know what it was. I feared not being taken seriously—by my readers, by an amorphous "anyone." I worried that people would believe my opinions to be influenced by my mental illness. I was fearful that people would not believe me because my perception of the world is off. I felt what is called "social stigma," and a lot of it I internalized.

I felt the stigma that most neurodivergent people feel all the time. We worry that we are not going to be believed in all areas of our lives. For example, we grow anxious about being believed when we seek medical care, as Dr. Kyle Younger explains in his chapter in this book when he struggled to find a mental health care provider who was a Black man like him. As he writes, "I was concerned that I would not have the therapeutic bond I needed if I worked with someone unable to draw upon similar experiential references." Younger knew that a white therapist would likely struggle to believe his experiences, and he did not want to deal with that disbelief in a caregiver setting. He describes the damage to his mental health that being Black in academia causes: "On a personal level, the microaggressions are taxing on my mental health. They cause anger, frustration, sadness, and even self-doubt." Would a white mental health care provider understand his experiences and know how to help him? Most likely, no. But, as Younger points out, there is a dearth of Black therapists: they compose only 4.1% of therapists in the United States. Sharing his own experiences plus research in this area of intersectionality that is typically ignored by those who study mental health and neurodiversity brings to the fore the importance of intersectionality in fighting the stigma of neurodiversity.

Other types of "vulnerable faculty" (as law professor Meera Deo puts it) who take great risks when disclosing their neurodivergences include contingent faculty who have poor job security (Deo 2022). During my 10-year higher education career, I chose to keep my neurodivergence a secret. First, I was a teaching assistant and graduate student. Then I was an adjunct on a year-to-year contract teaching multiple classes across multiple campuses, hauling my pregnant body down the highway and across different divisions at different universities. I gave birth to a premature child and then to a second child not 2 years later. During this time, my husband was getting his business up and running. Back then, our health insurance was my health insurance. I pulled in half of our income. If I had lost my job, we would have been fucked. But, gradually, things changed, and I was vulnerable no longer. I was free from the mask I had to wear on my campus.

But that freedom also stemmed partially from my inherent privilege: I am a white woman in a heterosexual marriage. I was able to quit my job because I had built up a reliable income outside of higher education, my husband's job started providing health insurance, and his income had grown so that I could lean on him as I built up my new career. Skallerup Bessette also points out how privilege intersects with neurodiversity in her chapter for this book when she describes having "a job that is flexible enough that I can work from home" (so do I) and excellent insurance (same here). Skallerup Bessette specifies all of the pressure points where neurodiversity and society crash into one another, frequently tragically. This is not to say that her life or mine have been easy; they have not. But we do have an ability to be generous and outspoken that others do not.

While using my newfound freedom to speak out back in 2014 and in the decade since, I have learned this: Speaking out is not about being brave. It is about stepping up to the plate because others cannot.

*   *   *

Stigma researchers typically divide stigma against neurodivergent people into three types: public stigma, internalized stigma, and institutional stigma. Public stigma is the stigma we encounter day-to-day, when someone says, "OMG, my boss is *so bipolar*" or when you first watch *The Big Bang Theory* and realize that there is nothing funny about how terribly everyone treats Sheldon and that he is the butt of the joke, not the hero. (The show's creators swear he is not autistic. We autistics know when someone is trying to dodge a question.)

Internalized stigma, or self-stigma, comprises what we think of ourselves, even if we are not aware of it. Just as Ronnie K. Stephens describes in his chapter, I sought out a screening for autism late in life because my children were diagnosed with it. (Dixie L. Burns describes in great detail how hard it can be to get diagnosed with autism as an adult.) Finally diagnosed as autistic in my early 40s, I felt immense relief. All of the awkwardness and plain *wrongness* I had felt for decades finally made sense. I thought, "Now I can finally drop the mask." But I was wrong. It took years and lots of therapy to stop getting angry at myself for saying "the wrong thing" or feeling embarrassed in social situations. Self-stigma is perhaps the most insidious of them all because we are harming ourselves, and, to fight it, we must wage an internal battle.

Institutional stigma includes things like poor insurance coverage for mental health care compared with physical health care—or the question on the TSA PreCheck quiz that asks whether you have ever been an inpatient for mental health care, using mental health care as a proxy for likeliness to commit violence (Pryal 2016).

Stigma researchers know that one way to fight stigma—all stigma—is to read stories by other neurodivergent people. For example, celebrities' accounts of their own neurodivergences not only help bring about institutional change but also help a lonely kid dealing with internalized stigma. Personal narratives of neurodiversity like the ones in this book also help. When a neurodivergent graduate student or adjunct picks up this book, that reader will feel affirmed. When a neurotypical provost or dean or even a chancellor opens its pages and sees how their neurodivergent community members suffer because of the institutional ableism they condone, changes begin.

The most important work that a book like this one can do is save lives. No, I am not exaggerating. Because when someone picks up this book and sees themself in someone's story, they understand that they are not alone. Being not-alone can give someone hope, encourage them to seek help, and show them they *can* make it through whatever suffering they are experiencing.

Because of this book, they just might step back from the ledge.

Over a decade after I wrote my first essay about stigma, disclosure, and higher education, I am holding an entire book full of stories by neurodivergent faculty willing to kick stigma in the face by publicly revealing their status as neurodivergent and their struggles with their mental health. These writers have all done something incredibly generous for those who cannot speak out.

It is true that our society does not treat people like us well. But if you are in a position to be generous, I beg you, be generous. For every voice like mine and those in this book are hundreds who cannot utter a word at all. Share your own stories if you can. Enact better policies if you have the power to do so. Speak out for those who cannot.

Introduction

REBECCA POPE-RUARK AND
LEE SKALLERUP BESSETTE

WHILE HIGHER EDUCATION is becoming more adept at supporting student health, the neurodiversity and mental health of faculty and staff have long lived in the shadows, at the edge between what is respectable and what is eccentric, what is "normal" and what is not in the academy. For students, neurodiversity and mental health challenges have been dramatically on the rise for decades (Abrams 2020; Anderson 2020a, 2020b; Gray 2015; Rutter and Mintz 2019). Even prior to the pandemic, universities and colleges were making moves to care for students by beefing up their counseling services, adding administrative positions in charge of student well-being and increasing student programming around physical health and mindfulness, while at the same time often dealing more openly and directly with student mental health crises and suicides.

But what of efforts addressing faculty and staff neurodivergence and mental health? Writing in the *Chronicle of Higher Education*, Emma Pettit (2016) highlighted how campus services for students were on the rise but were not available to faculty. And while faculty may have access to insurance benefits or an employee assistance program, the stigma surrounding being discovered to be someone who needs mental health care is often enough to keep faculty away from using these services.

After all, higher education is a culture of achievement, competition, reputation, and excellence, almost at all costs—not really conditions that set the stage for success for individuals with mental health disorders or neurodivergence. At best a neurodivergent faculty member or one with a mental illness might be labeled idiosyncratic, at worst, a "nutjob." These faculty and staff face stigma and perhaps even active hostility in their departments and institutions, if they make it that far. Seeking treatment and accommodation can be a minefield in our critically overloaded care system for fear of being "found out," stigmatized for having a "disordered brain" in a culture that values only logic and reason, or even losing one's job.

Mental illness, chronic and emergent, is not a rarity in higher education, just as it is not rare in the general population of the United States. According to recent research, 26% of adults in the United States above the age of 18 will or do experience diagnosable mental illness, and almost 10% will experience depression in their lifetime (Johns Hopkins Medicine 2024). Many people who live with mental health disorders deal with more than one at a time, as anxiety, depression, attention deficit hyperactivity disorder (ADHD), bipolar disorder, and obsessive-compulsive disorder frequently prove to be comorbidities. A 2019 study conducted by AdvanceHE showed that 36% of the 6,000 respondents had been treated for depression, anxiety, or both (Williams 2019). This study also found that only 14% of 150,000 postgraduate researchers who responded said they had *not* experienced medium to high levels of anxiety (Williams 2019). A 2017 report from the Centers for Disease Control and Prevention stated that 2.2%, or over 5 million, adults in the US have been diagnosed as on the autism spectrum. And these studies were done in the years prior to the COVID-19 pandemic. Recent research has called the underrepresentation of faculty with disability and invisible illnesses "stark" (Brown et al. 2018, 985, cited in Mellifont 2023, 866).

But these are just impersonal facts. They do not call to mind the real people behind the statistics, those whose lives you interact with every day without thinking about how you might affect them: the department colleague with borderline personality disorder; the librarian with autism;

the English professor with severe anxiety; the faculty developer with ADHD. In some ways higher education is the perfect place for these colleagues to be given its autonomy, its flexibility, and its rituals. It makes perfect sense. But in other ways it makes no sense at all. The rigid structures of the promotion process, the focus on collegiality and professionalism, the role of the rational mind above all else—our brains are our currency. When they do not work like everyone else's, where do we belong?

In this collection we explore these questions and dualities through personal narratives. The book's title, *Of Many Minds*, speaks to the multiplicity of minds you will find in higher education, not just fully logical and rational ones but many variations and flavors. As such we bring two flavors to editing this collection and to writing this introduction. Next we will individually share our lenses for approaching our work as coeditors before setting the stage for the narratives you will read in the sections that follow.

Lee's Perspective

If there is one thing that became clear to me while editing this collection, it is that higher education is a trap for neurodivergent people.

It is not the *only* trap, but it is one of the more seductive. Structures that support flexibility, encourage and reward hyperfixations, provide clear guidelines, and have some degree of tolerance for, let us call it, *quirkiness*. The masking is seemingly easier, at least at first, and fuels a neurotypical view of ourselves: If I can just do these things, I will be accepted in this space.

In reading these first-person accounts of neurodiversity in the academy, the pattern of the trap that higher education set for all of us becomes clear: We were rewarded at various points of our academic journeys, and things often seen as weaknesses or detriments were celebrated. But slowly or all at once, the pressures of structural ableism, conformity, and our own internalized ableism have caused us enough harm that our mental health has suffered.

I am not the only one who notes this phenomenon. In discussing autism in the academy, Irish writes, "Some people who gravitate toward faculty careers clearly fit into the broad criteria of 'gifted'—high academic achievement being a common trait. Giftedness and autism share a number of behavioral characteristics, and the presence of giftedness can obscure the fact that an individual is also autistic and mask the particular challenges and difficulties that gifted autistic people face in higher education" (Irish 2023).

In speaking with a friend who was recently diagnosed as having ADHD, they noted that the number of people they knew in academia who had ADHD was way more than it should be given the percentage of people with ADHD in the general population. Academia does seem to attract a disproportionate number of neurodivergent people, which makes sense, until it does not. The narratives in this collection make plain the levels of ableism in higher education and the toll such takes on someone's mental health.

I am struck by what Damian Mellifont says in his essay "Ableist Ivory Towers": "It is ableism that presides where a neurodivergent academic might still be of the mindset that they have to endure unfair treatments in higher education because worse experiences might be had elsewhere" (2023, 880). This, too, is a part of the trap; academia at least makes gestures toward inclusivity, even if it is still a system seeped in ableism. Aimée Morrison (my podcast cohost) put it thusly when it comes to seeking accommodations in academia: "University accommodations bureaucracies proceduralized a series of biographic mediations that split disabled people in two, differentiating disability and ability: an illness, diagnosis, impairment, deficit, or lack that can be 'accommodated' formally on the one hand, and, on the other, an underlying, non-disabled person with a required, standard (that is to say, superhuman) ability to achieve excellence through rigorous and independent self-application in the usual ways" (2019, 699).

Or, as she and I often put it in our podcast, "How can you have ADHD/be autistic? You're so successful!" To hold a position anywhere in academia is viewed as a success, and therefore any diagnosis of neurodivergence is in many ways negated.

This negation, the pressure to mask, to conform to ableist expectations, has a real impact. This book, rather than focusing on mental health first, initially looks instead at neurodiversity and the personal stories of neurodivergent faculty and staff in higher education. The two are linked, but what many of these essays show is the ableism of the academy toward those who are neurodivergent, which has a negative impact on mental health. It is an important distinction; I (Lee) am not depressed or anxious because of my ADHD but because my ADHD had been masked for so long and maligned by higher education. Many of us were denied a diagnosis of our neurodivergent condition due to our mental health, rather than understanding that our mental health was directly related to our lack of a diagnosis.

Masking, to a certain extent, is *easier* in academia. We can paper over our neurodivergent selves, hide the toll it takes on our mental health, and keep coming back for more:

> Many symptoms of mental and emotional distress among faculty can be masked by the very tendencies toward overwork and perfectionism that academia selects for, and faculty are often encouraged in this very behavior. The messages many receive from mentors and colleagues about how to manage the stress, anxiety, and pressure associated with academic life often involve some version of "work harder," "focus more on productivity," or "be grateful for the flexibility of academia." In other words, such concerns are often minimized. . . . Faculty often feel obligated to work at the neglect of self-care as being perceived as lacking constant productivity can affect annual reviews, promotion portfolios, and other opportunities within and beyond the home department. This sort of policing of behavior can also directly impact mental health and harm relationships. (Johnson and Lester 2021)

This is an ableist approach to being a professor, where someone's neurodivergence or mental health is not a consideration when given advice on productivity or "balance." Overwork can be an effective mask, however, albeit a temporary one.

The pressure (and the masking) starts from the beginning of our academic training: "Rigorous training programs select top-tier students who have much of their identity tied up in high performance and achievement. Such identity is greatly challenged during the course of training and into the career span; the demands of academia consistently confront individuals with their own shortcomings, promote unrealistic upward social comparisons, and drive high standards of approval" (Bira and Evans 2019). A comorbidity to ADHD is rejection-sensitive dysphoria, which can be devastating in the kind of competitive environment higher education sets up for faculty in particular.

Morrison writes, "Disability identity itself is rooted in story. . . . Disability identity also offers the potentially radical opportunity for rewriting a life story in the face of a new diagnosis" (2019, 694). Each one of the chapters in this collection reflects a person at a different point in their journey with their diagnoses, in rewriting their life story; there is no one linear path to come to accept one's own various conditions, let alone accept higher education's unwillingness to accommodate neurodiversity. No one in this collection is a mental health professional or an expert in neurodiversity, but we have all had to become experts in our own selves and situations. For some of us, situating ourselves within the larger conversations around mental health, equity, inclusion, and neurodiversity has provided structure and guidance. Others of us are still finding our voice and our space. Some authors have enough distance to be able to articulate advice. Others are mid-process and still raw from revelations and asking themselves: Who am I when the mask comes off, and is there still a place for me in academia?

Rebecca's Perspective

> Who tells the stories [of mental disability in higher education]? Who is privileged or deprivileged through the telling? In what ways might we want to change the stories we are telling, the ways we are imagining the proper place of the disabled mind in college? Indeed, do we even know what it means to have a disabled (unsound, ill, irrational, crazy) mind in the educational realm, a realm expressly dedicated to the life of the mind? (Price 2011, 2)

I have been struggling to write this introduction for months now. How can we do justice to the stories told in these pages? What gives us the right or the privilege to preface them, to belong with them, to categorize them, and to tell you what you should do with them? The narratives in this book are heartbreaking, powerful, compassionate, empowering, and disheartening all at once. They talk about the depths of mania and depression, the harsh realities of bipolar disorder and ADHD, and the wide range of experiences along the autism spectrum. The storytellers are colleagues and peers, parents, grandparents, neighbors, community members. They are us. Maybe they are you. One thing we all share is our connection to the culture of academia, one that "can contribute to, exacerbate, or even instigate mental health challenges for faculty and students alike" (Johnson and Lester 2021).

Academia is a place where intellect is valued above all else and where conditions are not necessarily supportive of individuals' mental health. Housel (2023) cites a 2020 Cactus Foundation study that supported past research on workplace factors that negatively affect academics' mental health, such as "long working hours, workplace bullying, pressure to perform, [and] inadequate workplace policies around work-life balance, harassment, and other areas, among other factors" (14). Housel then adds to this list, including "perfectionism; workplace bullying; social isolation and lack of peer support in academia's competitive culture; the output-driven culture, control, and surveillance in today's neoliberal educational, political, economic, and social environments; job insecurity and dismal job markets; pressure to be always available (especially for online instructors), and never-ending workloads that collectively increase workplace stress and mental health challenges" (15).

Yet, even with all these cultural factors influencing academics' mental well-being and ability to be successful, neurodiversity and mental illness among academics is often (subconsciously and consciously) viewed as a personal weakness or character flaw by those with neurotypical brains, stigmatizing those seemingly unable to "handle" the never-ending rigors of research, service, and teaching demanded of them even with accommodation (Housel 2023; Meluch 2023). Dolan (2023) states that neurodiversity and mental health disorders are invisible disabilities that refer to "a mental, cognitive, or physical impairment that is not easily detectable by an observer. This is a crucial distinction when we are examining the impact of disability in the profession that considers intellect to be a person's most valuable asset" (690). She further argues that faculty in her study believed, regardless of how capable they were, that disclosing their invisible disability "could prevent them from advancing their scholarly careers and might lead to their unwarranted alienation from the academy" (690). Bira and Smith (2019) note in their discussion of the stigma surrounding mental health disorders in higher education that these "'invisible wounds' . . . show themselves in disruptive emotional and behavioral patterns, which are unfortunately often attributed to personality flaws, work ethic deficits, underachievement, and health issues." What benefit is there, then, in telling these stories and, perhaps more importantly, for our contributors to share their own stories?

As Lee discusses above, it is too easy and all too familiar for neurodivergent individuals and those with mental health issues to internalize the stigma and ableism around them and to assume that they are the problem, not society or higher education itself. Mellifont (2023) argues that "disability stigma in the academy is far from harmless. . . . [It] can have a silencing effect . . . [and] under an ableist shroud of silence, opportunities for neurodivergent academics to gain access to mental health supports (where needed and wanted) might be diminished" (878). As this stigma is internalized, it creates "feelings of isolation and shame" (Pryal 2024a) that further separate the academic from the rest of their colleagues and profession. Participants in a study by Smith and colleagues (2022) found that stigma was "multi-layered [and] insidious," leading academics to grapple internally with whether revealing their neurodiversity status or mental health disorder was worth it for fear of "being discredited" or excluded from academia altogether, and they often internalized shame, which kept them from seeking necessary help (21–23). And as higher education "creates and nurtures ableism and individualism among scholars," Dolan (2023) finds it ironic that "universities appear to ignore the warning signs that ableism could ultimately put their institutional health in jeopardy. And as a consequence, a large number of professors regrettably live with the fear of being perceived incompetent" (693). This is where the work of story comes in.

Brené Brown frequently reminds her readers that we are wired for connection and for story. It is evolutionary. I am not telling you anything you did not already know. I found my way to storytelling when in 2018 I experienced a life-changing bout of burnout and its relatives, depression and anxiety, from my privileged place of tenure at a liberal arts university (Pope-Ruark 2022). Telling the story of my symptoms, my diagnosis, my vulnerability as my mental health declined, and then eventually rebounded, probably saved my life, along with a very good therapist. Aimée Morrison (2019) says that "disability identity itself is rooted in story" (694) and that "diagnosis performs the affirmation of the 'realness' of the disability; it produces disability in a given instance as a scientific, objective pathological fact" (700). But she also argues that this is a "useful fiction" for the medical machine and a way for academia to silence people who do not fit into the "fully rational brain on a stick" model of a professor (700, 706).

The presence of my book on burnout, Lee's writing on ADHD and being a "bad feminist," and the stories presented in this book, along with so many others, shows Margaret Price (2011) to be accurate when she argues, "The abundance of stories indicates that mental disability is not now—if it ever was—a rare occurrence . . . for a diagnosis is in essence a story" (3). For so many of the authors in our collection, diagnosis was a turning point in our lives; a point when things finally made sense and clicked into place, when narratives shifted and more fully aligned with who we actually were, not who we did not know we were. And for many of our authors, this new identity that came with a diagnosis, many late in life, offered "the potentially radical opportunity for rewriting a life story" (Morrison 2019, 694). We hope this book offers the same or at least a fraction of that feeling to you as a reader.

Why narratives? A few of the stories in these pages are what we might call autoethnographies or scholarly personal narratives, to use Brookfield's (2017) term, with an added critique of the academy and somewhat of a literature review. Others are chronological narratives of a diagnosis story or a life or a career. Some are snapshots of lived experience. Many are stories that have been erased by the current rhetoric around medical diagnosis, accommodation, and wellness. Price

(2011) believes that "incorporating narratives of experience is one way to improve access to academic prose" (25) because in the medicalized realm of mental disability, "persons with mental disabilities are presumed not to be competent, nor understandable, nor valuable, nor whole. . . . The failure to make sense, as measured against those with 'normal' minds, means a loss of personhood" (26), what Catherine Predergast calls "a rhetorical black hole" (198). Who are we when we are not allowed to speak our truth or believed to be rational enough to deserve the right to speak in an institution that values the brain and logic and rhetoricity and the dialogic above all else? Who has the right to mediate that positioning?

Here we give our contributors back their rhetorical voice and allow them to share that voice in their own way, without heavy editing to fit whatever normative standard academic editing might typically require. This is one reason I have so greatly appreciated Lee's coeditorship on this project; where my instinct as a professional writing and rhetoric professor was to add subheadings everywhere and "fix" grammar and structure, hers was to let the voices shine through however they needed and wanted (okay, I still added subheadings). And she was right. Our contributors claim their own stories of diagnosis, coming into being with a new understanding of self, of overcoming, but also of giving up, of doing just enough to get by and stay healthy. And they do so in language that is sometimes strained because their experience is strained, or convoluted because their lens is convoluted, or run-on because that is simply how their one of many minds works.

Part of allowing them their own voice is allowing them to choose their own terminology for their conditions. Personally, I identify my depression, generalized anxiety disorder, and past experience with burnout as mental health disorders, but contributors also use words like "neurodiverse," "mental illness," and "mental disability." The literature gives us varying definitions and rationales for using different terms. For example, Katie Rose Guest Pryal (2024b) defines "'neurodiversity' as an umbrella term that encompasses a variety of mental disabilities, including developmental disorders." Price and Kerschbaum (2017) use the term "mental disabilities" in their report on faculty to exemplify "conditions including depression, anxiety, mood disorders, personality disorders, autism, and other illnesses or disabilities affecting mental function" (5). And in earlier work, Price (2011) looks at the difference between using the term "mental illness," which she says "introduces a discourse of wellness/unwellness into the notion of madness," and the term "mental health," which implies that a person can be cured of mental illness by the medical system (12). Allowing our contributors to use the language they are most comfortable with is another way in which we return their rhetorical agency and positionality.

I end my portion of the introduction with this quote from an article by Johnson and Lester (2021), who remind us that "mental health is not simply an individual concern. All participants in academic life bear some responsibility for perpetuating harmful and damaging policies, practices, and norms of behavior, even if only by accommodation or inaction. It is incumbent upon all of us not only to attend to our own wellbeing but also to work actively to enhance and protect the wellbeing of others around us."

We hope the stories in this book contribute to this work.

Collection Framework

We have multiple purposes for this book, not the least of which is to give space to neurodivergent faculty and staff to share their stories in their own voices. If we help someone feel less alone in their own journey, then we have accomplished something important and valuable. But we also want to create space in organizations for difficult discussions around ableism and exclusion; each story is a case study where we can ask: How could we do better for someone like this within our department, unit, or institution? There is still so much to do, so much that can and should be done. Consider this collection as another way to start the conversations with your colleagues.

Each contributor has placed their trust in us, the editors, to help them tell their stories, and now we, the editors, are trusting you, the reader, to approach this collection with a spirit of openness and generous thinking, to borrow from Kathleen Fitzpatrick (2021). We are your friends and colleagues. We are instructors, staff, parents, partners, caregivers. We are all accomplished. We are also all neurodivergent and want to write, and tell, our stories.

The first section, "Coping and Masking," examines the various ways that neurodivergent faculty and staff have hidden or mitigated their differences in the face of ableist pressures, along with the freedom and challenges that come with unmasking. In *Unmasking Autism: Discovering the New Faces of Neurodiversity* by Devon Price, masking is defined as "any presentation of the disability that deviates from the standard image we see in most diagnostic tools and nearly all media portrayals," as well as any time "suffering wasn't taken seriously for reasons of class, race, gender, age, lack of access to health care, or the presence of other conditions" (Price 2022, 6). While every story in the book shares some extended narrative of masking, those that make up this section focus particularly on the impact of masking and unmasking.

Catherine J. Denial examines the internal and external pressures to mask mental illness, asking if accommodations, in some cases, do more harm than good and in fact encourage continued masking. David Dault shares his story of finally bringing his whole, unmasked self to work and in particular to his students when teaching. Emily Van Walleghen is able to ask the question, once the mask comes off, of whether working in higher education is what she really wants and whether it is good for her health. Jim Luke narrates what happens when your physical health dictates that the mask must finally come off. Each of these essays follows a common narrative, but each person comes to a different conclusion, following a different path, which can help make sense of your own masking or the masking of your colleagues.

The second section concerns itself more with the higher education structures that are harmful (and rarely helpful) for neurodivergent staff and faculty. These essays are a harsh look at academia, and while most of the contributors finally find some reprieve, it is in spite of the systems in place, not because of them. Most felt isolated and disconnected from the institution and community and upon trying to reach out found they still had to fend for themselves. This shared experience of systemic exclusion should be a wake-up call as to the harm the institution is causing.

Jorden Cummings writes about never fitting in in academia and how breaking free of that expectation allowed her to become healthier and more productive and fulfilled. Shannan Palma notes, and this observation could be for everyone contributing to this collection: "Assumptions often become the biggest barrier for me in a work or social setting. Both science and culture normalize general-to-specific neural processing, imposing cause and effect narratives on individual behavior that will rarely if ever be entirely accurate for anyone and that become tangible barriers for those of us whose brains function fundamentally differently. What fascinates me is how often these narratives serve ideology rather than humanity."

Robert Perret shares his struggles of trying to find a place within academia, while Darcy Gordon interrogates intersectional identities and expectations around mental illness, with a call for more vulnerability. Rounding out the section, coeditor Rebecca Pope-Ruark looks to understand how the structures of higher education work to limit her success given her anxiety disorder.

The final part, Stigma, examines the different ways in which the contributors have felt, experienced, or moved through the stigmatization of their conditions in the academy. Western culture in general does not look kindly on those who are neurodivergent or have mental health disorders, but neoliberal academia as a bastion of logic and rationality further shames those individuals with its deeply ingrained ableism.

In her story "No One Brought a Casserole," Melissa Nichols explores how an experience with a troubled student exacerbated her own mental health conditions, and she shares how her colleagues reacted, or did not react, to her situation and how she was ultimately stigmatized out of a job. Ronnie K. Stephens then explores his troubled relationship with formalized schooling and working within the structure of higher education and how his personality disorder makes forming relationships and, especially, networking very difficult. Coeditor Lee Skallerup Bessette, in her essay "Don't Ask Me How I'm Doing," examines the stigma surrounding being a "bad parent" and "bad feminist" as she manages her ADHD while trying to support her children as they navigate their own struggles with neurodiversity and mental health disorders. Dixie L.

Burns narrates her journey from childhood through today as an autistic academic who received a late-in-life diagnosis that had an impact on her ability to both understand herself better and encouraged her to become an advocate for neurodivergent students at her institution and beyond. And, finally, Kyle Younger examines stigma and the intersection of his identities as a Black man in academia with bipolar disorder II and generalized anxiety disorder.

The book ends with a bonus chapter from Katrina Swinehart Held, "'It's Okay to Be Human' and Other Lessons Learned under My Desk," in which she parallels her own struggles with advice for how faculty members can better engage neurodivergent students and those with mental health disorders in the classroom and in daily interactions.

We encourage you to think about the various ways you can engage with, think about, and discuss the narratives in this collection as ways to better understand neurodivergent colleagues and those with mental health concerns, as well as the role higher education and individual institutions play in supporting, or not supporting, our thriving. These narratives make excellent case studies for reading groups or working groups by making the clinical personal. Many of the emotions shared in these chapters along with lived experience should give us each pause as we think about behaviors and interactions with our own colleagues. How would you react to a colleague in one of these situations? How can you reinforce the structure and attitudes that lift up this colleague, rather than those that leave them feeling shame and stigma? How can higher education just simply do better to be more inclusive and supportive?

COPING AND MASKING

Cope: to deal effectively with something difficult
Mask: to conceal from view

ONE

For Those Who Do Not Love the Archives

CATHERINE J. DENIAL

AT THE HEART of a historian's work sits solitude.

This is a claim that needs some contextualization. Many historians collaborate on projects, practice oral history, draw on deep-seated community relationships, and/or do work hinging on the various publics found at museums, historic sites, and national parks. Yet for all historians, our research requires us to spend at least some time in archives, special collections, and libraries in order to analyze and contextualize the people we study (Reyes 2019). Many of us spend time alone when we write, entering into solitude to craft sentences and paragraphs that communicate our thoughts, whether those words are meant for other historians and educators or members of the public who might pick up a newspaper, or read a blog, or watch an informative reel on Instagram. Much of the working of the profession presumes solitariness. There is a professional expectation that historians should move anywhere for a job or a fellowship, the terms of each giving little consideration to the support networks that sustain us. And academic work often creates solitude—for example, by asking contingent faculty to work at four different campuses per semester to secure something like a living wage.

The platonic ideal of a historian's solitude is captured by the stereotypical vision of a professor in American culture. In television, films, stock photographs, and AI-generated images, such a person is a comfortably affluent, older, white, cisgender man who works diligently in an office crammed with books. His office is often illuminated by shafts of sunlight that spill in through large picture windows, and his every movement causes dust motes to dance. Sometimes, if a historian, this professor ventures out to the archives. There he examines letters, diaries, account books, and newspapers, perhaps indulging in a little paleography in order to discover new secrets. The reading room in which he works is always outfitted with wooden shelves and tables and trim, and it is peaceful and perfectly quiet. We are rarely granted a peek into the interiority of that professor's mind, but nothing about the professor suggests turmoil. The professor thrives on solitude and quiet and whatever deep thoughts he is thinking about the past.

I am not that professor; I do not have that mind.

Disquiet

When I enter a reading room, I carry not only the stories and theories and questions that will help me with my research but the effects of complex post-traumatic stress disorder (C-PTSD). PTSD is caused by trauma. It can occur after a single harrowing event like a car crash, a violent crime, or a sexual assault, especially if the victim does not feel supported in the aftermath, has someone pour doubt on their account, or is unable to process their feelings with people they trust. But for some people, trauma is not about a single event but rather about pervasive experiences—long-term abuse, racism, misogyny, queerphobia, prolonged combat, poverty—that undermine their basic sense of safety and dignity. That is when PTSD earns the prefix "complex."

PTSD is rooted in the human urge to survive terrible misfortune. The dump of adrenaline into our system when we are injured or terrified provides us with physical and mental strength. Stress hormones flood the body. In response we fight back, or we freeze, or we flee the situation, and sometimes we try to appease the person inflicting harm so they will stop what they are doing. All these things are human reactions to serious threats. We look to minimize those threats or escape by the means that make the most sense to us at the time—the stuff of sheer survival. But without the opportunity to process what has happened (or continues to happen) to us, those survival mechanisms can become maladjusted, causing us to perceive that we are always under threat and generating outsized reactions to everyday stimuli, like crowded spaces, loud conversations, stressful work situations, or movies, television shows, and books that contain approximations of the situations(s) that traumatized us to begin with.

This list is necessarily partial in that it is mine. I have been triggered by fictional depictions of assault; by congressional hearings for Supreme Court justices; by the sound of wind in a storm; by dreams; by something flickering in my peripheral vision; by a routine appointment for a visa application being canceled without anyone notifying me ahead of time; by the smell of hot tar on a summer's day. When I am triggered, my body and brain prime themselves to survive, sometimes by snatching away my access to my emotions so I appear cool and calm, or perhaps just grumpy, when in fact I am dissociating. I sometimes experience flashbacks in which I am immersed in the scents and sensations, the reality of past trauma as much as the reality of the present. Sometimes I am sensorially overloaded or deeply angry and frustrated without any obviously precipitating event, and it is only after hours or days have passed that I recognize the often innocuous thing that led my brain to string together associations until it summoned up fear.

Masking

A pervasive gap has always existed between me and the stereotypical calm, male, older professor. Setting aside my diagnosis, I am a woman, I was raised working class, and I am mid-career rather than close to retirement (if such a thing exists for any of us anymore). But more than anything, I cannot sit with the solitude of the archive for lengthy periods of time. My brain is accustomed to constantly scanning for danger, and failing to find it does not immediately stop me from looking for it. When my C-PTSD exerted its strongest grip on my life, I knew the world to be so unpredictable and dangerous that I often could not leave my house, much less travel to another state to dig through the collections of any particular historical society. My second-year review on the way to tenure was marked by my department's observation that I had made no progress on a research agenda, and this was not okay. I had not told them about my diagnosis because I was certain I would be fired, as surely no one would want me near students when I could not stay rooted in the present. I worked so hard every day to show up and teach all my classes; it was an unbearable struggle to write my lectures and get out of my front door. I masked—desperately presenting an appearance of mental health and/or neurotypicality to others so I would be accepted and stay employed. I did everything I could to be the right kind of professor while scared that it was an impossible task.

Masking is a reasonable reaction to the serious stigma that surrounds mental illness in many countries, including the United States, where I live. "The most prominent stereotypes surrounding the mentally ill presume dangerousness, unpredictability and unreliability," wrote Wulf Rössler in 2016. Individuals who are mentally ill not only see, hear, and absorb this stereotyping but often internalize it, leading them to worry that they are, in fact, as unstable as the publics around them believe them to be. The effects are serious. In a 2019 poll, the American Psychiatric Association discovered that roughly "half of workers were concerned about discussing mental health issues at their jobs. More than one in three were concerned about retaliation or being fired if they sought mental health care."

Academia is a workplace like any other. In a 2017 survey of "a large group of self-identified faculty with mental-health histories across a range of institutions in the United States," Margaret Price, Mark S. Salzer, Amber O'Shea, and Stephanie L. Kerschbaum found that 34% of respondents had never disclosed their illness to anyone at work (Price et al. 2017). Individual stories back up this raw data. Writer Sejal A. Shah wrote in 2019 of her decision not to reveal her own bipolar disorder. "I was in my mid-twenties and studying in an MFA program when my mind began to slip," she wrote. "But I could never admit this. I had a public self who appeared to be well. I had students. I intended to work in academia" (Shah 2019). Shah kept her secret through graduate school and into the early years of her career: "I looked normal; I passed. Would my career have turned out differently had I been willing to come out (for that's what it felt like, an emergence into a world that might not accept me)? I was certain the stigma of having a major mood disorder would have hurt me professionally" (2019). While experiencing deep postpartum depression and both bipolar and obsessive-compulsive disorders that had yet to be diagnosed, historian Ariel Mae Lambe (2022) "completed and defended my dissertation and started my tenure-track job, the modicum of energy and sanity I possessed spent entirely on those efforts. The idea that I needed to stay silent to protect my career compounded my general adherence to stoicism."

I masked until my second-year review made it impossible to keep my secret any longer. I told my dean and my department about my diagnosis and still remember how visibly one colleague recoiled from me, saying "I don't need to know any of that!" My dean told me I needed therapy at a time when mental health parity did not exist in the insurance industry, and I could not afford to pay someone $150 an hour while I earned $40,000 a year and could barely pay my debts. I did talk to my primary care physician about antidepressants and took them diligently, but because they were ill-matched to my person and situation, they had little effect.

This, then, was my professional unmasking—or at least it was the first of many. People who had power over my career encouraged me not to ask for an extension on the tenure clock, which might have helped me to get well, and no one suggested any accommodations to aid me. I was told quite directly to respond with grit and get my work done, so I put my mask back on and did as bidden. My situation seemed to disappear from my colleagues' awareness; more than one of them put me in instructional situations that triggered me so badly I could not teach for days.

But I got tenure at the same time as the other members of my cohort, and I published a book. I did so at a tremendous cost, my utter exhaustion leading to suicidal ideation. In that moment, at least, I knew telling others was the key to my wellness. I called my therapist and told my friends. I did not, however, tell my colleagues.

A Claim upon Wellness

After the Affordable Care Act passed and I found a therapist who specialized in eye movement desensitization and reprocessing, I started a new, uneven path toward healing. My psychiatrist shook her head in disbelief at the prescription I had been taking for years and found a mix of medications that gave me energy and renewed determination. My campus roiled, as so many did in the 2010s, with protests focused on sexual assault, and I grew more comfortable telling people I had C-PTSD if it modeled something about survival to my students. But I still tried to be That Professor—the dispassionate one, the focused one, the one for whom solitude and research were beloved companions. And in 2018 I applied for and won a fellowship to spend four weeks at the American Philosophical Society (APS) in Philadelphia to research the early 19th-century history of the Ojibwe people within its collections. The notification that I had been selected as a fellow stunned me. I felt triumphant. I had a fellowship. I was going to sit in a reading room and chase clues about the past with the best of them. I was *well*.

I was not, on reflection, well, but I was hopeful. I had learned as an international exchange student in 1992 that moving to a new city provided the dizzying opportunity to reinvent oneself. Whenever I dislocated myself from the familiar, I walked into situations where no one knew my stories, and I could invent myself over and over again. As I planned my summer in Philadelphia, I could see myself, in my mind's eye, cheerfully walking between my temporary apartment and the APS, soaking up the novelty of a city where I would flourish. I would thrill to every discovery I made from every document I read; I would buy flowers at the farmer's market; I would see art and visit museums and relish every large-city opportunity I could. I steadfastly set aside the fact that my entire body burned with my desire to stay at home.

Philadelphia did not turn out to be an escape. Instead, it was persistently noisy, especially at night when the garbage company would come to empty the 7-Eleven's dumpster. I did not know my way around the city and felt, as a consequence, that nowhere was safe. The first night after I arrived enormous protests took place against President Donald J.

Trump's immigration policies in the streets around my apartment, and while I absolutely agreed with the point of the protests, I was also knocked off-center by the chaos and noise. My own perception of my environment aside, things went wrong and increased my sense of anguish. My bank refused to credit my fellowship check to my account for fear that it was fraudulent, leaving me without any money for 10 long days. A key on my laptop broke, forcing me to send the machine away to be fixed and complicating my efforts to stay connected to friends through email and chat. In the reading room at the APS, calling up box after box of documents to examine, my mind churned with self-recrimination. The quiet there, the sage-colored walls, the here-and-there murmurs of the archivists all acted as a backdrop for the spiraling of my thoughts. You are scared. You are needy. Why are you here? You are getting nothing done. What a terrible mistake you have made. What a terrible mistake you *are*. I masked this as best I could by projecting confidence, by trying to talk back to the anxiety in my head, by spending fewer and fewer hours in the reading room over time, and eventually by drinking too much in my apartment at night.

I wrote in careful ways that did not do justice to the depth of my feelings about this situation in my public-facing blog (Denial 2018):

> Most of my time is spent alone in the library, in one-way communication
> with people who are thoroughly dead. Their words and ideas fascinate
> me, but it takes a particular kind of focus and attention to read them for
> hour after hour. . . . For all intents and purposes, working in the archive
> means it's down to me and the dead people, and even on the days where
> I find something particularly significant in the record, there are few people
> who can appreciate with me why it's so special. Significance requires
> context, and archival work is done almost without context, except for
> that which we bring with us in our own heads.

I was alone. Friends in New Jersey invited me to visit, and for two days at a time, on a couple of weekends, I felt relief. But for days upon days, I spoke only to the staff at the checkout counter in Target or the person at the reception desk at the APS. Solitude, the very marrow of my profession, was poisonous to me, and this was a conundrum I could not solve. I kept a private journal during my trip, but I masked even there. Looking back through it now, I can see that I was desperately trying to find something good to hold onto—the blueberry muffins at the farmer's market; the single, beautiful wineglass I bought for myself at West Elm; the English-themed pub across the square. But I barely mentioned my misery, that I longed for home and community with my whole heart and felt desperate and caged.

Hope for the Unruly

On my return home, I sought accommodations for my disability because I was at the end of my tether. It was hard, nevertheless, to know what I should ask. In the United States, the Americans with Disabilities Act dictates that individuals must be able to perform the "essential functions" of their jobs and that all accommodations must be "reasonable." As Margaret Price (2011) argues in *Mad at School*, it is tricky to know exactly what this means when it comes to mental illness:

> For example, what if a professor who has agoraphobia or panic disorder must miss classes on an unpredictable basis? Does the burden lie upon him to find a substitute, no matter how short the notice or distressing the situation that gave rise to the absence in the first place? If he does find a substitute, is that an adequate replacement for the work expected of him? What if he cannot be physically present, but periodically holds classes online? Can we still say that his teaching is good? Good enough? That it can be called *teaching* at all?

I ended up asking for permission to leave campus by 2:00 p.m. every day. It was an inelegant fix—it required me to project consummate capability in the morning but then allowed me to go home and collapse in the afternoon.

As I write, five years have passed since that fellowship in Philadelphia. I have continued to heal, albeit unevenly, thanks to therapy and coaching and the webs of friendship and mutual aid that sustain my life. But I am struck, as I shape these sentences, by just how much academics with mental illness are structurally rendered a problem to be solved, rather than constituting the impetus to critically reflect on the assumptions of "normalcy" that undergird higher education. As instructional designer Sarah Silverman put it in 2023 when talking about the requests she has received for tips for teaching neurodivergent students, "The best way to start is to figure out how normalcy is present and enforced in our classrooms or disciplines. . . . It's usually easy to identify where normalcy is present and causing harm, and not at all easy to undo it."

In my situation my accommodations perpetuate my masking; they do not create a workplace that questions its assumptions about what it means to be well, to do a good job, or to have a vibrant career. I have learned it is unlikely I will ever be the professor who spends a year at the National Humanities Center or the Radcliffe Institute, or even a month at the Newberry Library, because my support networks radiate out from the small midwestern town where I live and the home I have stuffed to the gills with color and comfort. Ableism renders some measure of professional accomplishment out of my reach. But this is not because of me—this is because my profession cannot countenance that dislocation and solitude do not serve us all well or make provision for a flourishing that is embedded, not separated, from community. As the poet Elizabeth Hoover (n.d.) writes about working in an archive, "A letter turns over to an empty verso, a blank my want tumbles into." The wants of so many people—safety, dignity, support, reimagination—*should* cause a collective reexamination of professional presumptions. How wonderful if the archive—and the classroom and the faculty meeting—could become disquieted by the unruly thinking of historians with my kind of mind.

TWO

To Be Seen as a Whole Person

Masking and Unmasking in Higher Education

DAVID DAULT

THE ISSUES OF MASKING, late-life diagnosis, multiple diagnoses, and "outing" myself to students and colleagues are my focus here. The context of the essay is my time in graduate school and on the tenure track in two different religiously affiliated university settings, as well as my observations about what has led to a contrast of outcomes.

The period when I was in my doctoral program was the first time I had access to consistent and affordable mental health care. Spanning from my late 20s to my mid-30s, this time marked an intense period of growth and recovery. It was also when I first became aware of the multiple diagnoses that frame my identity today. I now understand that complex post-traumatic stress, psychosis, depression, anxiety, and addiction have all played a part in my journey.

I entered the tenure track for the first time the year after I received my doctorate, and though I appeared to make progress "on schedule" on the outside, on the inside I was falling apart. This eventually manifested as a complete inability to write; not simply writer's block but a loss of typing and even longhand, swallowed in a thick flood of constant anxiety. I masked this from all my colleagues for the next two years and quit my position for a job in the nonprofit sector the year before I was scheduled to go up for tenure review.

Now, 10 years later, my recovery continues. I am once again on the tenure track, this time with a more balanced neurochemistry and a much stronger support system. Moreover, I have made the decision to be "unmasked" to my students and colleagues, offering them a more transparent view into the struggles and even the failings that I face in my daily journey of healing. The responses have been very supportive, particularly among my students, who tell me that in my modeling of a functional life with severe mental illness, they find resonances with their own experiences, strengths, and hopes.

Background

My mother and father divorced when I was eight. Prior to that, my home life was marked by periods of explosive domestic violence, including an instance of gun violence in which my father was wounded and hospitalized. After the divorce my father largely disappeared from my life for most of the rest of my childhood (we reconnected when I was in my early 20s).

My mother was a functional alcoholic and was polyaddicted to a number of prescription drugs. Throughout my childhood I experienced periods of neglect and periods of abuse. It seemed as if my mother had three distinct personalities: one was warm and loving; one was withdrawn and sometimes bordered on catatonic. The third personality was feral, paranoid, and often exceedingly violent. It was never clear, in a given moment, which version of my mother I was going to get. Her personality, and with it my safety and well-being, could shift in an instant.

To protect my sense of self, I began various forms of internal escape. Most acutely, I began dissociating in the fourth grade. By my fifth-grade year, I was regularly experiencing reality as if I were outside myself. It was like I was observing things happening to me but not engaged. As I moved into adolescence, this strategy expanded into escape in all senses of the word. I spent as much time away from home as possible to avoid confrontations.

I learned to hide my dissociation and to give the appearance of a normal child, but inside I was a wasteland. I have since learned the term "alexithymia," which means a difficulty in experiencing, describing, or expressing emotions. For all my adolescence and much of my early adulthood, this was my internal reality.

The other escape that presented itself was intoxication. I did not do much drinking in high school, but I did experiment with pills. When I got to college, I discovered that I could really hold my liquor. I found my place in a culture that rewarded binge drinking, and I got very good at it.

I continued these cycles of drinking, eventually to the point of blackouts, through my 20s and into my 30s. During the span of six years between the end of my undergraduate work and the start of my graduate studies, I continued to drink heavily. I got involved in a series of very unhealthy romantic relationships, worked a series of low-paying jobs, and mismanaged my finances to the point of bankruptcy. I knew things were not working, and I desperately wanted a way out, but I had no idea where to start or which direction to turn.

Trauma Response

There is a joke I heard once. Or maybe it was serious, I don't know, but either way I heard once that a professor started her lecture on the first day of class by asking the students, "How do you know your enrollment in seminary isn't simply a trauma response?"

I mention that now because my entry into graduate studies began with me enrolling in seminary, and I am absolutely convinced that it was, in fact, a trauma response. I had just lost all my money, and a serious relationship had imploded. In the months after the breakup and the bankruptcy, while I was putting myself back together, I guess you could say I found religion.

I had been an awful student in college, and my adviser had discouraged me from pursuing graduate studies, so enrolling in seminary felt like the longest of long shots, a true Hail Mary. I was ecstatic when I found out they would let me in. Suddenly, pushing 30, I was back in school. To everybody around me, I looked like a grownup, but inside, hidden from the light, I was a child. Rage, cheap beer, risky sex, and Percocet were my drugs of choice.

Here is something you need to understand: I have never had a hangover. I inherited that from my mother. She and I both had the physical ability to appear fully functional while we were blacked out and then get up the next day and start again. I even reached the point for a while where I was proud of my ability to seem prepared when I was hopelessly impaired. I seemed to treat it like a challenge. Or at least I imagine I did. I do not remember a good deal from that time in my life. That was what it was all about—killing off my memory and running from feelings I had no idea how to name, let alone handle.

As you might imagine, I got good at lying. I lied to everybody, including myself. I imagined I was this busy little beaver, toiling away at grand construction projects, when in fact I was just a cockroach, or maybe a dung beetle, scurrying around in my own crap.

I turned out to be a good student in seminary, though. I was good enough that I landed a spot in a doctoral program, along with a little bit of funding. On paper, at least, I seemed to be making something of myself. My deleterious habits, however, had reached an acute phase. Fellow students were telling me things I had said and done that I could not recall, and I had long since gone from being a pleasant drunk to being an irritable and increasingly violent one.

In the recovery community, we talk about seeing the bottom come at you. I know the night I saw mine. That is a story I do not tell, but in a moment of clarity, my addictions had my full attention.

First Diagnoses

I was lucky. I was in grad school at a major university, and for me that meant having access to mental health services for the first time in my life. I jumped in with both feet. By the midpoint in my program, I was doing individual therapy every other week, group therapy once a week, and a 12-step program twice a week. When I met the woman who is now my wife, we added weekly couples therapy into the mix.

What I want to communicate to you is that none of this—my recovery of my sobriety, my health, and my sense of myself—has been linear. I have come back to the question of "my diagnoses" again and again, each time with greater clarity and a more helpful narrative.

When I was a teenager and in my 20s, the only word I knew for what I was going through was "depression." That word was a blunt instrument. It named an area of my experience, but that area stayed mostly in the shadows.

I credit two therapists in particular with helping me in the long and tenuous work of reconnecting my words and my emotions. Alexithymia is obliteration; your reactions can be severe and explosive, but you can rarely explain why. More shadows. These two counselors ventured down into the darkness with a flashlight and a tool bag and helped teach me how (and also teach my wife to help support me) to begin to make repairs.

After a few years in therapy and recovery, my blunt self-description had acquired more detail. Along with depression, I was dealing with psychosis (my dissociation) and complex post-traumatic stress disorder. As I tended to my depression and got it more under control, I discovered new aspects lurking underneath its heavy fog blanket: severe anxiety and white-hot anger.

Wearing the Mask

This is what I was carrying with me when I entered my first journey on the tenure track. In addition to the work of finishing my doctorate, I had been doing this recovery work. A good deal had been unearthed, and some of my emotional apparatus had been reconnected to language, but I was a long way from health. I was in that stage sometimes referred to as a dry drunk, when you have stepped away from the rhythm of triggers and acute substance abuse, but all the underlying addictive behaviors are still in full operation.

I first learned the term "masking" in 2022, from reading *Unmasking Autism: Discovering the New Faces of Neurodiversity* by my Loyola colleague Devon Price. Price (2022) defines masking as "any presentation of the disability that deviates from the standard image we see in most diagnostic tools and nearly all media portrayals," as well as any time "suffering wasn't taken seriously for reasons of class, race, gender, age, lack of access to health care, or the presence of other conditions" (6).

Looking back now, this term describes what I was doing with my colleagues and students. I was expending a huge amount of energy keeping up the appearance of having everything together. I showed up, taught my classes, and met my professional obligations. I did not *look* like a recovering addict, a psychotic, or a survivor of trauma. Moreover, I did not dare show anyone (outside my family) that this was my daily reality. My terror at being found out added to my anxiety.

My wife describes those years to me now as an exhausted fog. I was present but I was not really *there*. It was taking everything I had to survive from day to day. My recovery became static, and progress became elusive.

During this period my anxiety became acute, and all my scholarly work basically ceased. I could no longer write because, every time I tried, my brain locked up in a white-hot flash. Colleagues would ask how things were going, and I would simply lie about my progress. I knew, however, that there was no way I would clear the hurdle of promotion. As much as I was hustling to appear normal and put together, fake it until you make it was not going to work.

After three years of this worsening situation, my wife and I had a very honest conversation. We agreed that we both needed to make some major changes if we wanted our marriage, and me, to survive. In 2013 I left the first tenure-track job, and we moved north to Chicago, where I started working in the nonprofit sector.

Unmasking

My family has been foundational to my recovery. One of the techniques my wife and I learned in couples counseling was reflective listening. This is a practice in which one of us says what we are feeling, and the other person's goal is to repeat back, as close to verbatim as possible, what the first person said without renarration or editorialization. The listener repeats the words of the speaker until the speaker feels they have been fully heard, and then the listener has space to ask questions or respond.

When this was introduced to us, the counselor said, "This will feel stilted and boring, but stick with it. It works." Every bit of that prediction has proven true in our case. Reflective listening is slow, stilted, and boring—and it has probably saved my life. Over the past 15 years of our marriage, it has allowed me not only to reconnect to my own emotions but also to learn to trust another person with the whole of my experience.

So much of my life has been spent hiding myself from others, or when I did dare to speak my truth, having that truth twisted into gaslighting and weaponized against me. Through this practice of reflective listening, I learned to rebuild trust in myself and trust in others. It became part of how we have raised our children, as well, so my entire family has become for me a laboratory for the rebuilding of trust.

In recent years I have returned to the matter of my diagnoses. I have learned to honor and better manage my anger. I have learned to be gentle with myself in the face of my anxiety. I have learned to anticipate and navigate my traumas and the triggers that arise from them. I have learned that regular sleep, exercise, and nutrition are priceless foundations for my continued mental health. With support, my depression and psychosis are currently in remission. Things are not perfect, of course, but I am sober today and have been for many days prior, and I spend a good deal of my life in touch with serenity.

Stepping away from teaching was good for me because it allowed me to take an honest appraisal of what I liked about academia and what was toxic for me. After a couple of years in Chicago, I started picking up adjunct work at various colleges and seminaries around the city. I feel incredibly blessed that in 2020 an opportunity opened for me to join a faculty again.

Unlike my earlier experience, this time I have endeavored to bring my whole self to this opportunity, which includes my journey to mental health. I began experimentally, disclosing aspects to my dean and certain colleagues I trusted. Over time this circle of trust has grown to include the whole of my colleagues in the department, as well as my students.

Our institutions do not make it easy for students or faculty to be honest about the places where we are struggling and recovering. In my own life, this led me to continue the hiding and habits of self-harm and even created a perverse reward structure for living in the shadows.

I know that I am extraordinarily privileged to be able to pursue tenure not once, but twice, in my career. I know how lucky I have been to have a career in academia at all. I also know that I have not overcome the obstacles I have faced alone. My recovery has been possible because I had access to resources, time, and a tremendous amount of love from those around me.

Now, as a colleague and a teacher, I choose to share my story. My journey and my recovery are part of my pedagogy. I have found that this openness has created space for others to feel welcome to tell their stories, as well. Moreover, stepping out from behind my mask has opened ways to speak with students about self-care and to practice the centering of care in the structure of my courses.

In the recovery traditions, we have a phrase: "Progress, not perfection." None of this is ever going to work perfectly. It is likely I am never going to feel completely at home in academia, or even in my own skin. Yet when I look back, through writing this, I can see the progress. My hope is that some of my experience will be of use to you as you make your own journey, masked or unmasked. Know that I have faced some of what you are facing, I am in your corner, and I am cheering for you.

[THREE]

Barely Passing

EMILY VAN WALLEGHEN

Depiction

The students sitting through my medical nutrition therapy class know nothing about my life outside of that lecture hall. Perhaps they wonder what I do when I am not teaching. As far as they know, I am a person who shops at farmers markets carrying an upcycled canvas tote and wearing a J. Crew cardigan enjoying the crisp breeze and fog-filtered sunshine. It would be logical to assume their nutrition professor buys only local, in-season produce, after all. They envision I later join my close-knit group of friends for oat milk lattes, avocado toast, and spirited banter.

In reality, avocados disgust me (it is a texture thing), and I have not been to a restaurant in years. Instead, I am wearing eight-dollar polyester pajamas and sitting alone at the kitchen counter awkwardly perched on an uncomfortable stool. I am eating artificially sweetened, excessively packaged yogurt with a plastic fork and surfing PubMed on my coffee-splattered laptop. The curtains are drawn because the sunlight is exhausting. I vaguely recognize, yet ignore, that I am cold and leave my fan running for necessary background noise. I will not talk to anyone all day if I can help it.

After a battery of neuropsychiatric tests and a "formal diagnosis" of autism at the height of the pandemic and well into middle age, I was not only isolated from other humans but left questioning if I still counted as human. Now, with the return to "normalcy," I question both my desire and my ability to keep up the facade. Do I feel like I am a failure because I really want the life my students imagine for me, or is it that I have been conditioned à la allistic social norms to believe that I need to hide?[1]

Deliberation

I suppose it is difficult for me to come up with any even semi-intelligent and/or well-considered answers because it is complicated, and I do not have any expertise whatsoever. All I can do is relate my N-of-1 personal experience. My fear is that my writing will serve as an autobiographical case study and my warped self-analysis simply exhibit A of a curious, yet unrelatable, other. Or worse, my word choice, the context I provide, the window into my thought process will document my clear inability to fulfill my professional responsibilities.

Writing about my experience should also be rooted in a solid understanding of what autism *is*. The problem is that the meaning depends on who you ask, and there are a lot of opinions,[2] which is why I am still unsure whether I should embrace it or ignore it altogether. And, despite my best efforts, I still have only a rudimentary understanding of the complexities, so I am certainly not qualified to come up with a definition on my own. Given that I actively sought out a diagnosis, however, it seems I am endorsing it as a condition, or at least something that can exist simultaneously as a construct and condition.

With the pandemic-induced intensification of my otherwise inexplicable behavior, finding a reason for why I had, for example, showered at *exactly* 9:14 p.m. for the last *year* became imperative. Or why I ellipticaled (ellipticated?) for 62 minutes and 30 seconds (63 would be tragic) *every* morning. Or, to revisit the yogurt, why strawberry was clearly a flavor *only* for breakfast, and raspberry was *never* to be consumed before noon.[3] Although I fully understood that these rules were not rational, they made perfect sense in my head, and while I always hid them from the outside world, I never deviated from them. I needed a logical explanation for why I illogically dictated how I lived my life, and determining if it could be attributed to a specific etiology felt necessary.

But lacking an autism definition also means I cannot predict the potential implications of an autism label, and I can see why one might question the decision to risk acquiring it. All I can say is that, as for probably many people, lockdown for me became a venue for introspection within the context of overwhelming aloneness. Amid the stress and urgency of pivoting to teach into a Microsoft Teams abyss from my bedroom was also a new self-awareness stemming from the absence of anyone other than myself to learn more about, I suppose. Habits (rituals, if you buy into the autism vernacular) became more ingrained as there was no reason or opportunity to interrupt the sameness, and I could not escape myself. I eventually realized that each day was the same as the next not because it had to be but because nothing in the outside world was forcing me out of my rigid routine.

One of the advantages of my faculty position is access to health insurance that is both (relatively speaking) affordable and comprehensive, and the reality is that I am incredibly fortunate to even have the option of pursuing a diagnosis. Uncertainty is a difficult state in which to exist, and the unfairness of a health care system where it is disproportionately cost-prohibitive to pursue definitive answers is maddening. In retrospect it seems a bit twisted that although employment in academia is exactly what provided the means for the diagnostic evaluation I wanted, it led me to worry that a consequence of the resulting diagnosis could be unemployment in academia.

Diagnosis

I was evaluated by a clinical psychologist who cut no corners, and the process was unnerving and seemingly endless, some of it expected and some not so much. While my episodic memory of much of the testing itself is only still partially accessible, I do have a comprehensive report sent via encrypted email a few days afterward for corroboration. Part of the assessment still firmly ingrained, however—probably because the purpose was a perplexing mystery at the time—was to measure my ability to recount a verbally conveyed story. My result? I scored in the fifth percentile. The fifth. Given my perfectionist tendencies, this was kind of soul crushing in that it provided objective evidence that I cannot live up to my own expectations for myself. So, of course, for self-preservation purposes, I immediately went to work on shifting blame. And the recipient became my illustrious diagnostician.

First, the story was asinine, and I was not warned I would need to recall it. It was about . . . well, if I could not recollect it immediately after the fact, I am definitely a poor historian now. Something with a grandfather and a truck and buying bananas. I think. Anyway, the point is I would have remembered it in all its pointless detail if I had been told in advance I would be required to recall it. I made it through school forcing myself only when I knew I had to, but I sure as hell never scored in the fifth percentile on anything.

Second, the physical environment was set up for sabotage by distraction. The psychologist's office was a typical bland, beige space with the predictable drop ceiling tiles and fluorescent lights, but it was outfitted with giant executive-esque highly polished dark-stained furniture that I could not figure out. But more importantly, the excessive shelving was chock-full of his framed family photos: the kind where everyone is wearing matching polo shirts and smiles, posing in a perfectly manicured suburban backyard.

I do not have a family. Or the ability to smile on command. Or a yard. Or even a polo shirt. Although we were roughly the same age, having earned our respective doctorates long ago, what we did with them in the ensuing years was painful for me to contemplate. He had a highly accomplished career and the kind of normalcy I will never achieve. I struggled with the day-to-day tasks necessary to function and maintain gainful employment and had little else. How was I supposed to pay attention when he was rubbing that in my face? When you are busy hating yourself, it is hard to multitask.

Other components of the testing I only hazily recall and that have now mostly melted together involved solving series after series of physical puzzles, but I do have results of my performance on the individual tasks, which I fully expected to see in the report. What I did not anticipate was the inclusion of the psychologist's behavioral analysis conducted as I thought and assembled. In other words, he was spying on me from two feet away. I failed to detect this prior to reading, after the fact, "[She] was also observed to engage in sensory-seeking behavior as she repeatedly ran her fingers back and forth along the edges of the thick plastic desk protector on top of the evaluation table."

True, but seeing this in writing was alarming because I *knew* I engaged in these behaviors all the time in *professional situations*, and I realized I was deluding myself by assuming that no one noticed. Now when I stand in front of a lecture hall unable to resist the compulsion to pick at my cuticles in response to the overwhelmingness of subjecting myself to public display, I am hyperaware. But have I changed my behavior? Absolutely not. I still do it every day. It is just now more disconcerting because I know I am not hiding it. People notice. My students know.

The report ended with the final blow of the recommendations based on the exhaustive evaluation and "severity" of my autism. Among other action items, the "plan of care" included therapy/counseling to "focus on improving eye contact, voice inflexion, and affect; improving conversational skills; reducing social anxiety; and reducing nonfunctional repetitive behaviors or routines" along with occupational therapy for "reducing sensory-defensiveness."

Given this information, how could I not doubt I am someone who should be in charge of *anything*, let alone of providing a quality education to college students? If I now had "objective" evidence of my inhumanness, why on earth would I be trusted and paid to teach capable humans? Being myself is a disqualification from the position.

Disclosure

Although my ability to fulfill my responsibilities has not changed, I now monitor myself more meticulously and therefore have more opportunities for self-criticism. And I feel less competent because of it. I cannot help but wonder, then, if disclosure would also lead to closer surveillance by my superiors at work, looking for mistakes that could be interpreted as a decline in performance. Am I setting myself up for poor annual reviews and denial for reappointment?

I do not think it is even debatable that higher education is a business. At my institution the importance of increasing student numbers (and revenue) is the messaging from all levels of administration. Performance-based budgeting is a $%#@&,[4] and at the departmental level, the primary determinant of workload allocation is the number of students in a class, not the actual amount of time it takes to teach said class. Simply put, what matters is how many students I teach rather than whether I actually do a good job at teaching those students. The increase in quantity has to affect quality in some capacity, or it would not be sustainable. But doing just good enough is not an option for me, not only because I am insecure and seeking approval but because providing individual student attention gives me a sense of purpose and helps me make it through another miserably hard day. I want everyone in my classes to get it.

The result is that I am constantly on the defensive against the teaching *volume* and a workload that is unmanageable for me. And academic culture does not value complainers. The message is that if you cannot handle it, it is because you are not working hard enough. Sink or swim. The expectation is that working overtime and volunteering to do more is what the team players do. Asking to do *less* and being told I am already not doing enough makes me feel like a jerk for even raising the question. If excuses are just a sign of laziness, it seems easier to accept the hand I have been dealt. Pointing out a diagnosis that would just be perceived as a weakness does not seem worth it.

I think things would be different if I had applied for and began my current position with a diagnosis. More than 10 years into it, however, means a lot to contemplate, and my capacity for making decisions is extremely limited. Post diagnosis I view myself through a different lens, as someone operating from an inherent *deficit*, and I have no reason to expect anyone else not to do the same. No error can be overlooked but instead becomes a sign of disorder, of existence on an entirely different plane and an inability to understand or relate to the neurotypical experience. And because through this lens I have lost trust in my own capabilities, I am left with more questions about the professional implications and what I can accomplish in academia and in an allistic world in general.

Of course, all this overthinking and internal conflict is based on the perhaps misguided assumption that disclosure is actually a decision I must make. In reality it may have always been glaringly obvious to everyone else, and I am just decades late to the party. It is quite possible I am not as good at covering up as I think I am and that more evidence than just my bleeding cuticles is unquestionably implicating.

For an educator, communication skills are obviously vital, and outside the classroom, writing probably comprises the majority of communication work, so it seems like an apt example, and I will circle back there. I used to think of writing as a safe place where I could carefully plan appropriate responses that correctly conveyed the message I wanted to send. I could Google any idiom or figure of speech to ensure proper usage, and with the luxury of time to edit myself, I actually felt confident in my ability. I am not confident anymore.

Instead, now all I can see is the (perhaps characteristic) avoidance of contractions and convoluted sentence structure not only in professional writing but in the most casual emails. And beyond the misused formality and syntax, what exactly does my writing reveal about my idiosyncratic thinking? Part of my tendency to overexplain and leave no s p a c e can be ascribed to a long history of exposure to contrived scientific writing conventions in which you have failed if you have not managed to weave in the phrases "vicious cycle" and "future research is warranted," but part of it is also . . . me. No one will ever describe my writing as elegant, but is it blatantly pathological?

Desire

And then there is the issue of whether my diagnosis really matters. Regardless of my success (or lack thereof) in hiding all of this, the worst thing that could happen is that I would lose my job and all future prospects of working in academia. But assuming I have the choice of continuing to work in my current capacity, is it really in my best interest in terms of both my mental and physical health? Despite my nagging self-doubt, I know I *can* do this. But *should* I do this? Do I keep doing this because it is a good decision or because I am incapable of making the decision *not* to do it?

My worry about how I am perceived is not new, and the fact is I have spent a lifetime covering for myself, although I only just recently realized that. At work I have managed to show up in a different semipresentable sweater each day, but underneath I have been wearing the same ragged T-shirt circa early grad school for a week straight. When it peeks out, I beat myself up, and I do not think I will ever get that negative self-talk out of my head. It is constant, and the nature of my job is decidedly not helping me accept myself.

In fact, in at least one situation each day I feel decidedly *less than*. Still fresh in my mind, for instance, is a recent meeting where handling uncomfortable conversations and feeling discomfort in general was a topic of discussion. The consensus among everyone in attendance (other than myself) was that an uncomfortable space is something one should reframe to explore and inhabit and learn from. I have not nor will I ever have the capacity to consider my discomfort a fortuitous opportunity for self-growth. And I spent the rest of the meeting kicking myself for lacking the sophistication to do anything about it for the past 10-plus years other than . . . destroy my cuticles.

Every semester gets harder and each class more draining and stressful such that I am now convinced that the only way I stay standing and semicoherent is because my vasovagal and fight-or-flight responses cancel each other out. At some point, however, it is inevitable that I will either collapse to the filthy industrial carpet behind the lectern or take off running. . . . I just do not know which. Regardless, it seems evident that I need to stop trying to keep this up. On the other hand, if this is the only way I have ever functioned, can I, and should I, change that now? Are my rituals and reclusiveness in fact simply coping mechanisms? Escapes from the overwhelming world? Things to be managed and corrected according to my "plan of care"? Can I learn to be a person I am not?

Humans are social animals and all (or so I am told). If I should be social, it really would not behoove me to give up on teaching and find a work-from-home desk job where I would have no reason to ever leave the house.[5] An adult would learn to adapt, continuing along the same track and working toward achieving defined career goals. But why is that the status quo, and why should I abide by it? If I am wired in such a way that aloneness and routine really do make me happy and the only reason I feel bad is because society tells me it is impossible to live the way I do, maybe quitting is the correct decision. I operate in this job as if it is a job, not a career. I just try to live through the day to day and ignore the rest.

The reality is that even if strategizing professional advancement is beyond my bandwidth, I make up for that lack of deliberate planning and ambition with 100% dedication to doing the best I can in my teaching and for my students. Despite my frustration with the system, I accept my responsibilities and I do still care, deeply. And in the end, I think that is more important than the (many) social missteps. The message somehow gets across. Despite my paranoia I am not, in fact, in any imminent danger of losing my job. Feedback from my students is overwhelmingly positive, and my department chair acknowledges and even values that. It is just me who cannot. And, in all honesty, spending each day navigating exactly how to demonstrate caring is exhausting.

Denouncement

When it comes down to it, I cannot shake the sense that I am only observing the world that everyone else lives in. I do not have the access code, and no one will give it to me. There are no clear answers to any of this, at least for me (obviously), and certainly no clear path forward. Yet, at the same time, I do not think it is possible to remain in the in-between. The longer I stay here, the blurrier the line separating being who I am from faking who I am gets, confusing me even more. What I want and what is best for my life is so tangled with societal expectations in my brain that I do not know where one ends and the other begins. As isolated and alone as I feel in all this, however, I do recognize that my struggle is not unique. If sharing my inner turmoil can function as something useful in the outside world, putting it out there seems like a *human* responsibility. All I can hope is that this thinking out loud is a start to . . . *something*. I do not know what it looks like at the finish line, but I guess I will find out. Wish me luck.

NOTES

1. First described in this context by Andrew Main (Zefran) as a (clinical condition) counter to autism. "Allism," accessed November 26, 2023, https://www.fysh.org/%7Ezefram/allism/allism_intro.txt.

2. For example, commentaries on articles acknowledging differing and evolving definitions criticize the conceptualization of the variability in these definitions. Samuel J. R. A. Chawner and Michael John Owen, "Autism: A Model of Neurodevelopmental Diversity Informed by Genomics," *Frontiers in Psychiatry* 13 (September 2, 2022), https://doi.org/10.3389/fpsyt.2022.981691; Darko Sarovic, "Commentary: Autism: A Model of Neurodevelopmental Diversity Informed by Genomics," *Frontiers in Psychiatry* 14 (January 24, 2023), https://doi.org/10.3389/fpsyt.2023.1113592.

3. This is kind of untruthful in that it is only the tip of the iceberg. And also does not acknowledge that I navigate a *sea* of these icebergs every day. And end up stuck. #shackletonexpedition.

Here is the full rundown:

A.M. permitted flavors: aforementioned strawberry, blueberry, peach, lemon

P.M. permitted flavors: aforementioned raspberry, mixed berry, cherry, vanilla

Notice there are exactly four in each category? Yeah, that's intentional. But *plain* is allowed all day long! See how flexible I am?

4. Summarized nicely in this Nicolas Hillman, "Why Performance-Based College Funding Doesn't Work," accessed November 26, 2023, https://tcf.org/content/report/why-performance-based-college-funding-doesnt-work/.

Or, for a peer-reviewed publication: J. C. Ortagus, R. Kelchen, K. Rosinger, and N. Voorhees, "Performance-Based Funding in American Higher Education: A Systematic Synthesis of the Intended and Unintended Consequences," *Educational Evaluation and Policy Analysis* 42, no. 4 (2020): 520–550, https://doi.org/10.3102/0162373720953128.

5. One also might ask why I do not stay in academia but do research instead. First, in my experience that is not a thing. Most academic researchers still have teaching responsibilities, and even if that was not the case, you cannot just change tracks. It would cause the entire bureaucratic administrative system to implode. But pretending for a moment I could, it is, in my humble opinion, a huge misnomer that working in a lab is a good fit for someone with control issues and limited social skills. This is why after two (arguably failed) postdoc appointments, I left research. I am *so* not cut out for it.

FOUR

Ripping the Mask Off

The Body Knows What the Mind Denies

JIM LUKE

FALL SEMESTER 2021 was ending and along with it my four-month sabbatical. It was my first commute to campus in nearly two years. I have a long commute—over eighty miles—but I have always enjoyed it. It was my wife's and my solution to the two-academic-job problem. She does not enjoy driving, so we live near her university. Me? I have always loved highway driving, so for the 20 years before the pandemic I made that drive most days and loved it. I often did my best thinking and planning behind the wheel. It calmed me and helped me focus. It was often inspiring and even energizing. But not anymore. I was too fatigued to think or focus anymore.

I was returning from meeting with my faculty sabbatical mentor, a good friend. The handbook I had promised as my sabbatical work was only an outline and opening chapter. I was afraid Human Resources (HR) would demand to be repaid the sabbatical when I could not deliver the book. My mentor assured me that it was okay and that I had over-promised in my proposal. What was worse than my fear, though, was the sense of failure and frustration at having failed—again—to complete a large "real writing" project; a confirmation that I was indeed the quitter and lazy kid my early teachers had always said I was.

I arrived home by 2:00 p.m. but was fatigued, which continued for a few days. Then the email came. All full-time faculty were required to teach on campus, in person, at least one class in the coming semester, and my schedule had been changed accordingly. In three weeks I would have to start making the drive again multiple times each week. I did not have the energy. I could not. I began to panic. My recently retired wife made plans to drive me to class and have us stay nights in hotels. I reluctantly dug up the links to HR's Americans with Disabilities Act (ADA) accommodation request forms and contacted my doctor.

Hiding Physical Disabilities Until You Cannot

I am no stranger to physical disabilities. I am third-generation disabled, the child of a polio survivor and a tuberculosis survivor (with other disabilities). I learned long ago that it is best to hide invisible disabilities and not draw attention to visible ones—just manage things as best you can.

That principle was reinforced soon after I started work at my college many years ago. I developed debilitating neck and shoulder pain. My doctor identified the problem as the low, nonadjustable chair the college had provided. He wrote a letter recommending an ergonomic chair as an ADA accommodation. The HR department, after waiting weeks to respond and quibbling over the doctor's qualifications, reluctantly agreed, but it still took months for the chair to arrive.

Like many disabled, I have multiple disabilities, not just one big one. I have keratoconus, a visual impairment in which, among other symptoms, bright lights and glare create pain and distortions (Luke 2019). Even if I wear my special rigid gas-permeable contact lenses, which I can only do for limited hours each day, I am still very light-sensitive. When the school remodeled our office suite, they installed new LED lighting—a painful nightmare for keratoconus patients. I asked if my office could have different lights installed and explained why. I was given a firm "absolutely not." Given my earlier experiences, I left it at that. I just never turned the lights on, worked in the dark, and bought a small desk lamp. When you are disabled in higher ed, you make do. You do not push it unless really, really necessary. In 2022, I had to push it.

Other previously hidden disabilities included my extreme allergies and immune deficiency. For my nearly seven decades I have learned to manage asthma, hives, anaphylaxis, infections, and other respiratory issues. I carry an EpiPen. When the SARS-CoV-2 (COVID-19) pandemic struck in early 2020, I readily embraced wearing physical masks. I still do. Wearing a physical mask has kept me safe from COVID and other new infections for nearly four years now.

When Christmas 2021 came, I had avoided COVID, but I was not well. I had already been dealing with work stresses and lingering respiratory infections I had picked up before the pandemic while presenting at academic conferences in Europe and elsewhere. My lifelong immune issues had become more serious and complex, resulting in chronic fatigue and respiratory, neurological, and even cardiac symptoms. I was also developing cognitive difficulties and problems focusing. I increasingly had to limit many daily activities and alter routines that had long served me well, including the long commute.

Ripping Off the Metaphorical Mask

I filed my ADA accommodation request as soon as the New Year began with help from my wife and my doctor. This time, with my union urging a rapid decision, I was given accommodation to work remotely and teach asynchronously.

I was safe from virus exposure but disquieted. Then I realized that, with the ADA filing, I was now "officially" disabled. No more hiding my disabilities. It felt like having a mask ripped off—a mask I had no idea I was wearing. Further, I realized I had also been metaphorically masking my neurodivergence as well as my physical disabilities. I had been hiding my neurodivergence even from myself.

I have always known I was "different." Allergy and immune issues are hard to deny. My vision (besides the keratoconus) has also been very different from most other people's, although I did not discover that until adulthood. While I have long thought "my mind works differently," I never considered the full implications of that idea. I certainly never considered myself "neurodivergent." I am a child of the 1950s and 1960s. The word was not even used then!

As I researched my growing difficulties, I broke through decades of denial. Those daily routines, the ones I could no longer physically do, were not just personal quirks. They were essential for me to maintain a professional identity in workplaces where being neurodivergent— where having a "mind that works differently"—carries benefits but also creates many difficulties. My success in coping with the difficulties posed by my different mind enabled me to ignore or deny my actual neurodivergence. I had effectively masked my neurodivergence from myself until recent health challenges had ripped off that metaphorical mask.

"Masking" is a term widely used these days to describe many behaviors of neurodivergent people, both children and adults. It is a term borrowed from psychology and earlier from the theater. A typical definition emphasizes "the efforts and choices of individuals" to "hide or suppress their symptoms in order to conform to social expectations" (Stavraki 2023). It is, of course, a metaphor. Like so much discussion about neurodivergence by neurotypicals, it puts the emphasis on the individual as aberrant or deficient, someone to be fixed. The emphasis is on the individual and their "masquerade." Interestingly, we rarely discuss how our institutions mask or hide their reluctance to accept and accommodate neurodivergent faculty. The common use of the term "masking" ignores the broader social and institutional context.

I have grown increasingly uncomfortable with the terms "mask" or "masking" in the specific context of an adult academic neurodivergent. It leads us away from nuances, insights, and experiences that could help our students, faculty, and staff to live fuller, happier, healthier, and even longer lives. Since my realization of my own previously denied neurodivergence did feel like having a "mask ripped off," however, I will continue that usage as I tell my story.

Discovering Myself behind the Mask

Having to rip the mask off meant not only not driving but also not doing other activities I had thought were only idiosyncrasies. For example, as far back as middle school I began every day with an hour or more of reading the news while having a cola. By the time I graduated from college, I had a two-to-five-liter a day habit. It never occurred to me that I was self-medicating for attention deficit hyperactivity disorder (ADHD) with caffeine until two years ago when I had to quit caffeine because of health complications. I quickly found myself lost and struggling to focus. The ability to concentrate under pressure or produce on deadline has always been a strength of mine. I did not know it was a trait of ADHD called hyperfocus. I always thought ADHD simply meant hyperactivity and bouncing off the walls. I had been fidgety as a child, but much to my late mother's joy, I finally learned to sit still in middle school—when I started the caffeine habit.

As an adult I always assumed I could not have ADHD. When the mask came off, I mentioned to my best friend of 37 years, a professor and clinical psychologist, that I had discovered these ADHD traits that seemed familiar to me. I asked their opinion. They smiled and politely told me they had long suspected I was ADHD. The cracks in my denial grew. Once I could entertain the idea of my ADHD, I could see so many symptoms that fit: everything from my stimming/fidgeting and endless leg bouncing to complex symptoms like sleep disorders, disrupted circadian rhythms, and the way that highway driving calmed me down. I may have long ago given up outward physical hyperactivity, but inside, my brain never stops. I began to understand my complicated caffeine-fueled rituals for what they delivered: the ability to manage my focus each day. I could see how much effort I expended to maintain my professional identity as a highly productive scholar and academic. Once I began to understand ADHD, particularly from the stories and lived experiences of other ADHD academics, my own life, my struggles and successes, made so much more sense.

In much the same way that my uninformed and unexplored stereotype of ADHD enabled me to mask my identity from myself for so long, so, too, did my uninformed and unexplored stereotype of dyslexia. I always thought dyslexia simply meant "reverses letters" and "can't read well." Decades ago a close friend, a professional responsible for diagnosing dyslexia and vision issues for a five-county school district, told me I was dyslexic. He laid out the reasons back then, as well as the connections to my vision processing and how I had adapted my reading habits. Nonetheless, I simply ignored his diagnosis. My thinking went, "I am smart. I can read and read fast." My stereotype then of dyslexia did not fit the professional self-image I was developing. In that era I was a young star in corporate strategic planning circles with a growing reputation for innovation and seeing the big picture.

Those same interests continued as I transitioned many years later to a community college professor's life. In addition to my teaching, I developed an innovative Open Learning Lab at the college. I led the college's strategic planning efforts for a few years, and I spoke at conferences about big-picture concepts in higher ed. That work was fun and part of my identity, but it was also the prime source of stress that helped worsen my immune issues and that led to my mask being ripped off. I had not been trying to "mask" or camouflage my ADHD or dyslexia. I had just been trying to get my work done.

With more up-to-date research about dyslexia, I discovered my friend had been right all those years ago. I am dyslexic, but dyslexia is vastly more complex than I thought. I learned I read differently. Most folks read linearly, focusing on letters and words in sequence. I scan the shapes of words and phrases, my eyes moving rapidly back and forth and vertically on the page for a brain that is racing ahead and matching patterns. Layouts, contrast, fonts, and white space make dramatic differences to me. They determine whether I can zoom through with excellent comprehension or get stuck endlessly repeating the same parts of a line until I give up. Dyslexia, at the brain level, is far more diverse and complicated than popular stereotypes. I learned that dyslexia and ADHD often overlap, and the combination is associated with big-picture and systems thinking, including innovation—the exact qualities that had served me well in corporate strategy development but had proved to be such a mismatch in academic institutional culture (Taylor and Vestergaard 2022).

I learned that dyslexia is often involved with differences in visual, spatial, or speech processing. That felt extremely familiar. It resonated with why I feel so out of place in the writing-centric culture of higher education. My brain does not produce writing the way my neurotypical colleagues write and teach. It does not mean I am stupid or lazy, despite the microaggressive suggestions of many teachers, professors, and academic leaders. Understanding I had real differences—not deficits—in brain functioning helped me recover faster and avoid panic when an ordinary academic task blew up for me recently. I received the proofs file from the publisher for a book chapter I wrote. The editor had used Track Changes. The file had fonts, font sizes, colors, and a layout I could not change. It was not the best for me. My dyslexic brain was exhausted from coping with a medium, process, and task designed for a neurotypical brain. I was so frustrated and felt so stupid and ashamed that I lost it.

All my childhood trauma about reading and writing came back. I could think, but I could not talk at all, even to my wife, the safest person I know on the planet. I have now moved past that incident. In the past in my denial I would have internalized my struggle as stress while an internalized ableist voice said I am stupid, lazy, and not a "real" academic. Now I realize it is just part of the extra work necessary to be an academic when you are neurodivergent.

The Institution's Mask

I said earlier that I have grown uncomfortable using the term "masking." I emphasize that I am specifically considering the context of *adults*, faculty or staff, in a *professional* setting in *higher education*. In higher education everyone, including neurotypical folk, engages in some masking behaviors. Everybody works to present and maintain a professional identity or academic persona. But for neurodivergent faculty, it takes more to get and stay "in character."

The larger disability community has a term called "crip time." As explained to me by a wheelchair-using academic friend, it refers to the added time burden and the different experience of time disabled people face because of the barriers they encounter. The extra time a wheelchair user needs to plan, get to the car, load the chair? Crip time. The extra time to condition, monitor, and maintain my keratoconus lenses? Crip time. Maintaining and keeping a small emergency kit with me wherever I go? Crip time. Stimming and routines to maintain ADHD focus? Crip time.

We are all playing a role, a part, in this production we call higher education. The difference is that neurodivergent faculty experience a heavier burden of time, effort, energy, and emotion to play our roles in the way our institutions demand. I call that the crip tax. It is the extra burden, time, and energy we incur to fit into a work culture that does not make room for how our minds work. It is payable in time, stress, adrenaline, cortisol, and burnout. We are not trying to camouflage or masquerade. We are just trying to get the job done as we are told the job must be done. We can call this masking, but that metaphor has limits. It is too focused on the individual and not the institution, the culture, or the context.

Why Don't Neurodivergent Faculty and Staff Simply Ask for Help? Why Don't We Seek "Accommodations"?

The law requires a process for requesting ADA accommodation. A medical diagnosis and proposed specific accommodations are required (EEOC 2002). It is more focused on major physical disabilities than neurodivergence, though. Ironically, ADA law requires an "interactive process" to negotiate appropriate individualized accommodations. Only a form to complete and no one to talk with makes it not much of an interactive process. We know there is little chance of achieving a creative accommodation or a change to a process that might lessen the crip tax for autistics or those with ADHD or dyslexics or other neurodivergent faculty. One professor shared their ADHD experiences when I asked about masking. They said, "I don't try to hide it. I just don't see any point or benefit in mentioning it." The process is defensive, intended to protect the school from legal liability. But for the disabled and neurodivergent faculty, the process itself is another crip tax and a potential trauma trigger.

Every neurodivergent adult is different—from each other as well as from neurotypicals. We do not fit neatly into categories or labels, much to the frustration of many neurotypicals. One thing we nearly all share, though, is a history of trauma, even complex post-traumatic stress disorder (PTSD), the frequent result of our experiences in schools. The unique interplay of our particular trauma and brain development is a large part of what makes each of us unique. But it also makes us wounded. The wounds of my own complex PTSD are deep and easily triggered (Khiron Clinics 2021).

Asking for help does not feel safe. Who wants to ask for help from bureaucrats and risk being told they are not sufficiently neurodivergent or are too different to fit the defined categories based on a deficit/disease model? Who wants to risk hearing that they have failed to even be properly different? Who wants to risk being denigrated or triggering that PTSD?

If we are going to talk about the masking of neurodivergence in higher education, we need to talk about institutional and leadership masking. It is at these levels where school communications proclaim the importance of diversity, equity, and inclusion but fail to deliver. "Disabilities" will sometimes make the list, but it clearly means "minimal compliance with legal obligations" such as policing online documents for standard accessibility features. The official talk masks a reality where expectations make work harder and the culture less safe for those whose minds work differently. Our institutions' leaders wax eloquently about diversity, equity, and opening minds. The reality is a code of silence about neurodivergence in the academy. We do not discuss ADHD or autism or any of the other neurotypes among our faculty or staff. We do not listen to their lived experiences.

A serious physical illness forced me to rip off my "mask," engage with other academics, scholars, and researchers about neurodivergence, and reflect on my own brain and mind. I am better for it. My students are better for it.

I love the title of this book, *Of Many Minds*. To me that is what higher education should be. What it could be. The potential is so great, but to achieve our potential, we all need to "rip off the mask" about the realities of neurodivergence in the academy. Neurodivergent minds are not a problem to fix, a diagnosis to hide, or a deficit to "accommodate." They are richly different minds, nonstandard minds that enrich our institutions with creativity, insight, imagination, and different perspectives. We need to unmask our institutions and embrace conversations, safe ones, with all our many wonderful minds, neurotypical and neurodivergent.

HIGHER EDUCATION STRUCTURES

Structure: an arrangement of and relations between the parts or elements of something complex

[FIVE]

There Is No "One Path" in Academia

JORDEN CUMMINGS

WHEN I THINK about my first year on the tenure track, I think about constantly needing to push myself. I worked a few hours each day and then watched tons of television. I could drag myself to campus to teach but was exhausted afterward. I slept a lot. I loved working at home (and was productive there), avoiding my campus office as much as possible. I felt inadequate as a professor because I "worked so little." I beat myself up, mentally, all day long, about how I was a failure and always would be.

With the hindsight of 13 years of distance, I recognize much more in this experience: the extreme burnout I had by the time I finished my doctoral degree and started that job (with no time off in between); the reality that being unable to care for my chronic depression as a graduate student had worn out my body and mind.

But in that experience, there were some clues that this was how I work best. Some inner part of me cared for me, making sure I rested, pacing myself, and allowing myself to be home where I was productive and comfortable. Those were my early clues. . . . It is possible to be successful as a faculty member without working 60 hours a week and never sleeping. Who I am and how I work are not what we traditionally see modeled in academia. Academia tells us many lies, and one of its most damaging is that there is one single way to be successful (and thus productive, and therefore worthy). That lie tells us that we must grind 24/7 and that the quantity of our output measures our worth; that we are weak and unfit to be here if we do not hustle constantly.

I am a "success." I publish papers, hold grants, and am delighted to have won a teaching award. I am a research director and a tenured full professor. I have a book under contract, and people tell me my work influences their lives. I have led essential committees. I have graduated master's and doctoral students. I have a steady publication record and just received funding to build a new research cluster with innovative colleagues.

I am also successful based on my measuring stick (my values). I have balance. I start my mornings with tea and my journal. My identity is holistic and not just made up of my career. I work hard to value people over projects. I love working with graduate students because they say I am helpful to them. I have collaborators who I love to see and work with to generate cool ideas. I have hobbies. I make time for my loved ones. I pick up my kid from school every day.

At the moment of writing this, I love my job. For many years in my career, I never anticipated saying those words. My path has not been straightforward, and I consider myself a late bloomer—at least by academia's standards. One year into my full professordom, I am finally finding the meaning, engagement, and reward I always thought academia held for me. But it did not always feel like this.

My Unworkable Early Years

About three years into the tenure track, I had to ask my mother to come care for me. I had never done that before. My parents routinely drove to visit me in graduate school, heading straight south for eight hours from their home to the futon in the apartment I shared with my roommate. While there, they did all the generous things they had always done while I was at the university: took me shopping, stocked me up on groceries, cleaned while I studied, cooked real meals, encouraged a sleep routine, and enjoyed downtime with me, seeing local sights or watching movies.

Asking them to visit was routine. Asking my mother to be my *temporary caregiver* was not. But my depression—despite a good 15 years of experience learning to manage it—had become too much for me to function anymore. Those three years spent slogging toward tenure after the burnout of graduate school had only exacerbated my symptoms.

In addition to my depression (nothing new for me), I had started having panic attacks in our tense, contentious, and occasionally downright nasty department meetings. I dreaded speaking up but could not resist when processes or outcomes seemed unfair. The panic drove me out of the room routinely to briefly hide in my office or a bathroom. Or I stayed and doodled through the terror, telling colleagues who mentioned this that it "helped me concentrate." My physician refused to prescribe any medication for the panic attacks. I suffered. I eventually developed a bodily reaction to meetings I labeled "meeting ears." They would grow hot and turn red during the meeting. By the end they would be throbbing, burning, and red like lobsters.

This time my mother came alone, heading northwest on a plane from her home to the spare bedroom in my house. She took care of everything except my job. I was a windup toy version of myself: My mother would encourage me to get out of bed in the morning, cajole me to shower (against my wishes), feed me, and send me off to work (i.e., wind me up). I would use up all that energy putting on a smile and my energetic but bumbling professor persona at work, making people laugh, doing my job, and then driving myself home just as my energy wound down. I would eat something my mother cooked and go to bed. We would repeat the entire day the next morning.

I oscillated between feeling nothing to feeling utterly trapped in my life, believing that my specialized skill set left me no other career choices, and shattered that my dream job had been an illusion.

I spent these early years of my career, and many more to follow, assuming I was the problem. Because the path to success was *so evident* in academia (do research, publish, get grants, publish more, voila!), I internalized the idea that if I could not manage that without mental health problems or burnout, I must be broken. Sometimes this message came from inside my mind. Other times it was spoken to me by colleagues—even colleagues who seemed like friends. I constantly compared myself to other faculty and felt inferior because I assumed they needed less rest than I did, did not struggle with their mental health or physical fatigue like I did, and enjoyed working all the time when I, notably, hated the expectation that I would give my whole life to academia.

I concluded that I was not meant for academia. My depression demonstrated that I could not be a success. Yet I pushed forward, deciding to pursue tenure and using my resulting sabbatical to decide if I would quit.

Too scared to try any new approaches (in case they did not work), I used all my existing (unhelpful) coping strategies: pushing past my mental limits; ignoring my physical needs; engaging in zero hobbies or other interests; working all the time and at weird hours. There were a few glimpses of my future within there: finding a therapist I clicked with. I began to go to massage and physical therapy. I read about self-care. I vented to friends who loved me. But by the time I got tenure, I was broken by the journey.

If there was one way to do things, and I could not do it, where did that leave me?

Brian, My Inner Full Professor

After getting tenure, I began the slow journey of healing that has led me to today. I continued with therapy. I started hobbies and invested in friendships. I drastically reduced my work hours. I began working with a life coach. I obsessively journaled and read self-help books. I began pursuing the self-care research I had always wanted to do. I also discovered Brian, my inner full professor.

All this work focused on two big questions: What did I want my life to look like? What was getting in the way of that happening?

Much of this work happened in life-coaching sessions focused on my career: Where was it going? How could I work more efficiently to have more time for balance? How could I set boundaries and stop getting pulled so hard into what other people thought of me? Life coaching, in retrospect, used a strengths-based approach to pull the skills I already had out of me and gave me the freedom to be myself in my career. It gave me the wisdom to trust myself and helped me realize that I knew how I worked best and what I needed in my career . . . I just was letting other voices drown me out.

One voice, in particular, had a lot of power to sway me. It was not *my* voice in my head. It did not share my values. In one session, we pulled that voice out of me and named it for the someone else it was. This is how I met Brian, my inner full professor.

Brian is white, and he is old. He has been a full professor for so long that he no longer remembers what being any other rank is like. I picture him with bushy white eyebrows, a beard, and thick glasses. Brian was trained a long time ago—back when academics were all white, heterosexual, able-bodied men with wives at home to take care of every single thing domestic while the Brians of academia published papers (which was a lot easier when Brian was an associate professor and had an assistant to help). Brian firmly believes in publish or perish. There is not a project or a grant he will pass up. He believes that working evenings and weekends is required for academic success and that anyone who cannot do so is weak. He does not understand why anyone would not sacrifice everything for an academic career. Brian remains confused that I lack a secretary and must reconcile my purchasing card and submit my final grades. Brian does not value teaching except when he can mindlessly lecture for hours on end, only in an area of his expertise. To Brian, there is only one path to success in academia. And he likes to tell me that—a lot. Brian is always there to capitalize on my doubts to get me to work instead of rest or to take on another project instead of saying no.

I learned to recognize which thoughts belonged to Brian and which to me. I challenged whether Brian's suggestions were in my best interests or aligned with my values. I learned to separate myself from Brian, and we coexist peacefully now (except during grant season; he can still convince me I should apply for them all!) It took a long time to teach Brian that I know what I need for my success and that I am good; he does not need to worry about my progress and constantly tell me to work harder. Brian has learned that there are multiple ways to be successful in academia too.

As I let go of only listening to Brian, I was able to redesign how I approached my work to make it fit who I am. I stopped conflating my uniqueness with brokenness. I allowed myself to work at home, where I thrive. I made a million changes, some that worked and some that did not—but I felt safe exploring. I now understand the importance of context in our mental health and behavior (Hayes and Gregg 2001, 291–311). I was not broken—just in a context and using strategies that were not working for me.

Academia Is a Club Where I Do Not Belong (and That's Okay)

Along with feeling broken came the feeling of not fitting in. I realize now that a strong motivator for "doing academia" in a way that worsened my mental health was my desire to fit in. If I could only adapt and accept working all the time, the lack of sleep, the competition. . . . Then I would fit in, and all would be fabulous! For years I twisted and turned myself into various configurations designed to improve my fit with my department, institution, and academia (i.e., my context).

I withdrew, and I was drawn back in. I tried speaking less, and I tried speaking more. I tried new collaborations, some of which worked and some of which did not. I threw myself into any search committee I could, hoping we might hire more people like me (and we did). I chaired committees and undertook major administrative roles in my program and department, hoping to shape my context into something more workable for me. People who shared my values, like well-being and prioritizing good relations, thanked me for this work. Everyone else either ignored it or sometimes became an active roadblock.

I revisited this feeling of not belonging over and over. It was a pebble in my shoe. Nothing worked, no matter what I tried: I never felt like I belonged. Over time, as I took thousands of steps on top of that pebble while beginning to separate myself from Brian and experiment with more feasible ways to approach my career, I began to wonder about how to approach the pebble differently. What would happen if I stopped fighting this thought and considered that it might be true? What if, instead of trying to belong, I accepted that . . . I did not belong?

I realized it was true: I do not belong in academia. Because academia is a system that was not built for people like me (and many others). The more I thought about who academia was built for (white, able-bodied men of privilege who had caretakers at home), the more reasonable it seemed that I did not fit. The more I began accepting this, the more I stopped internalizing that not belonging was my fault, and the more I began to thrive.

I do not belong in academia for so many reasons: sexism, my values that disagree with exploiting and demeaning students, the incivility and bullying that should be unacceptable (but is an open "secret" that never will change), others who outrank me taking advantage of me, my disabilities, and my gender nonconformity. Sometimes this gross brew came all at once. I spent years in a role being treated as less than equal before I realized that gender (and rank) were being used against me. I did not want to admit I was being taken advantage of—this was my last bastion of trying to fit in. Once I finally realized I never would, I declared my time in that role over.

Realizing that academia is a club I do not belong to (and that not fitting in is okay) was a crucial first step toward accepting that my path to academic success might look different from what my inner Brian and others were telling me. When I accepted that I did not fit, my mind shifted. I stopped trying to become a conformity pretzel and instead began making my context practicable and seeking places I could fit, even within academia.

It frees up an unbelievable amount of mental space when we stop trying to figure out what is wrong with us (the answer is nothing!) and begin just . . . living as we are, actualizing who we are, and working in ways that are less what we "should" do and more what we want to do.

Using Play and Creative Hopelessness to Explore New Paths

Realizing I could stop trying to make myself fit and taming my inner Brian were both life-changing moments on my path to working outside the box and creating a context within academia where I could be successful, even with chronic mental and physical illnesses. I strove to adopt creative hopelessness, a concept from acceptance and commitment therapy that means realizing that we do not know exactly how to solve a problem but that what we have been trying is not working (Hayes et al. 2016). Adopting creative hopelessness opens the door to finding new behaviors to attempt with a lens of curiosity.

No longer worrying about "getting it right," combined with listening to my intuition about what might work best for me, led me to a space where I permitted myself to play with strategies—both for productive work and for balance outside my career. It opened the floodgates for me to ask myself what paths to success I would like to take. What worked for me? I experienced the empowerment and joy of beginning to structure a life consistent with my values.

Professionally, I turned my research to wellness and self-care for academics, helping professionals, and health professionals and launched Teach Me Self Care, where I disseminate this work.

Understanding that my body needs rest and that if I push it too far, I will pay the price back in spades, I center my days around getting enough sleep (routinely 10 hours a night—yes, it can be done) and pacing myself. It took years of tweaking to find what worked for me. I understand what my depression needs in any given week: lots of white space in my calendar to decide what to do flexibly and time to keep my physical space tidy and organized as well as a hefty dose of solitude balanced with regular time each week to catch up with loved ones and stay connected. I know what situations will make me anxious or overwhelmed (e.g., last-minute deadlines, specific committees, or combinations of certain colleagues) and minimize my exposure to them.

I have also recently learned that I am a multipotentialite with many interests, abilities, and pursuits (Wapnick 2018). Whereas I used to beat myself up moving back and forth from project to project, from diving into my teaching to starting a master's of education to applying for a new grant, I now recognize this is how I work best. Academia wants us to specialize. Brian was rarely thrilled with the diversification of my interests. But I grow bored focusing on only one thing, and learning about everything and anything allows me to be someone who integrates across disciplines.

Academia has spent years telling me that working in my way will lead to disaster. It has not. I am thriving. My mind and my body are getting the balance they need. I am at my peak (so far) in terms of my efficiency, productivity, and output and my sense of belonging with the colleagues whom I love working with. I feel joy at having created a life worth living.

This idea that there is "one path" to success in academia (combined with all the other ways that academia oppresses diversity, which is beyond the scope of this chapter) cripples the ability of so many of us to do our best work and enjoy our careers. I see this when I deliver self-care workshops to graduate students and early career faculty, in particular. There is so much fear that diverging from this prescriptive path (that our inner Brians tell us to walk, or else) will lead to catastrophe (generally in the form of becoming jobless), and people are unwilling to try. That makes sense! I was that graduate student, and I was that early career faculty member. Instead of taking the medical leave I needed and deserved, for example, I called my mom to deal with the rest of my life so I could still show up on campus and pretend I was okay.

Something amazing happens when we can drop out of the games of academia: We become ourselves, the people we were meant to be before academia twisted us into believing the lie that a very narrow range of acceptable behaviors and paths lead to success.

Over time I have learned how to manage my chronic depression. Occasionally, it rears its head, and the years since the start of the pandemic have been a struggle. Unfortunately, as is common with chronic depression (Monroe and Harkness 2005, 417–445), when my depression does reoccur, it is worse than it used to be. My depression can now manifest itself in suicidal thoughts or thoughts of self-harm. It continues to be mostly triggered by stress from academia. By critically evaluating the ways I succeed best, I have been able to take steps to minimize triggers and maximize approaching my career in workable ways.

SIX

But Why?

The Social Consequences of Boundaries as an AuDHD Person

SHANNAN PALMA

IN 2018 I WAS RECRUITED to apply for a job as the founding faculty director of a graduate program at a small liberal arts college (SLAC). Because I was not aware at the time that I was autistic, I had no idea how much my professional reputation hinged on having been in the same academic community for 14 years. I never realized how hard it would be to learn to navigate a new community or that my atypical body language and delayed processing frequently activate unconscious bias in neurotypical peers. I was used to a large private research university that had clear policies and organizational structures. I did not know how different the relational, do not-put-it-in-writing culture of a SLAC would be or how alienating my new colleagues would find my need for clear expectations and reporting structures.

I was also unaware of my attention deficit hyperactivity disorder (ADHD). I never considered how the expectations around rapidly responding to email and caring for students' emotional and mental health as a professor, administrator, and major adviser to 50-plus working graduate students while dealing with new course preps every semester would overwhelm my capacity. But as I became aware of these areas of challenge, even prior to diagnosis, I articulated my needs and boundaries as best I could.

In this piece, I will explore the ways in which ableist assumptions and resistance to formal systems break faith at all levels of the institution and encourage a culture where anxiety, paranoia, and trauma become weaponized instead of healed. In contrast, I will show how my current leadership role in a nonprofit start-up entails many of the same job functions and how having an inclusive, neurodiverse organizational culture allows me to excel at my job. I will close with recommendations for organizational practices to create environments where all can thrive.

Assumptions

Neurotypical brains trade detail and specificity for efficiency during development, hardwiring generalizations acquired from culture, family, and previous experience: the sound of the air conditioner is unimportant. Filter it out. The sound of Mother's voice is important. Prioritize it. Social rules gain use value because of what they signal about a person's place, power, and importance within the community.

Part of what makes my brain neurodivergent is that it works from the specific to the general. As such, my theory of mind—my ability to predict others' experiences based on my own—does not work with neurotypical people. Because of this, the world seems unpredictable. People act from all sorts of motivations that are intellectually understandable but not intuitive to me. I need the details of a situation in order to form a complete, nuanced picture. Over time, these pictures acquire layers and allow me to identify patterns. Once I have the pattern of a person's or organization's behavior, then I can use that as an attentional filter.

Anomalies in the pattern require attention and may signal a decision point. Once I understand them, I can react accordingly. If I fail to find a way to understand them, my nervous system reacts as though I am in danger. What to others may seem like an intellectual inquiry—"Why?"—is often a life-or-death question for me, experientially, regardless of the objective stakes.

*   *   *

In late 2017 I got an email. An acquaintance wanted me to look over the curriculum of a new graduate program and give them feedback. Our three-hour lunch resulted in them inviting me to apply for the position of the founding faculty director for the new program. I would get to build it from the ground up and implement the ideas and suggestions I had offered.

I hesitated. I had made a very intentional decision in grad school to pursue work in higher ed administration outside the professoriate. I loved my research, but my gut said that I was not meant for faculty politics. I do not get subtlety, and I need to know what the rules are in order to function. Faculty politics involves too many interpersonal dynamics that I do not understand. People are fragile and territorial in ways that make no sense to me.

But the work itself sounded fascinating and satisfying. I love teaching and designing curriculum. I was good at mentoring. I cared.

I applied. And I got the job.

The first six months were good. I brought my full self to work for the first time. I needed all of me in order to do the job. I did not try to make myself small. I did not assume that I was the problem every time people seemed frustrated or upset, both of which I had done in the past. I brought all my passion and directness to bear to advocate for the people and program I saw as mine.

It did not go well.

The culture of the SLAC was one of constant change. I can handle change and am very good at pivoting quickly, but I do that by maintaining a consistent narrative thread connecting the various turns. I need the handholds of chronology—we decided X, but now Y has happened, so instead we are going to do Z.

I need to understand the reason for the change in order to maintain the integrity of the overall patterns I use to function in general-to-specific culture. I need to know why. The reason can be as simple as the person in charge said so—I understand hierarchy. Hierarchy is a reason. But I need there to BE a reason.

I also need to know that I am not missing important information because my attention glitched, which (ADHD) is a thing that happens.

If you have ever been out in blizzard conditions, or read a book about farming in blizzard conditions, you may remember the old trick of tying a rope from the back door of the house to the barn. Farmers did this so they could hold on to the lifeline and use it as a guide to get to their animals in a whiteout, when the snow and wind made every direction look the same. They would hold on to the line and follow it wherever they needed to go.

Knowing why is my lifeline, my consistent narrative thread. It is how I settle the inexplicable part of myself that is constantly overloaded and overwhelmed by sensing and attempting to process everything, everywhere, all at once.

My brain does not automatically filter the world. I have learned to tune up or tune down my senses. I wish I could tell you how.

For example, about 12–24 hours into a camping trip or other outdoor adventure, I always experience a noticeable physical release. It is like a big portion of my operating system frees up for other tasks. I just feel lighter. No technology. No city noise. No confusing social rules. Just me, maybe a close friend or two, and the world. The world is not too much. I can handle just-the-world. I do not have to expend constant mental effort muting 90% of my perceptions when it is just me and the trees and the wind.

My attentional dampening field is not, I have learned, the same as a neurotypical attentional filter. It takes constant effort. And because I cannot turn it off or on again quickly, I mostly have to just leave it running 24/7, focusing on one thing at a time and hoping there is nothing I am actively not noticing that could threaten or harm me or someone else.

Because if there is, odds are I am not going to notice it until too late.

*   *   *

When I started the new job, I asked questions to understand. But my questions were met with what seemed to me to be inexplicable hostility. In retrospect I realize the administrator who had recruited me took my directness as an attack on their leadership. I am decent at recognizing social cues in a timely fashion when I understand them, but in this case I was oblivious, as at the time the administrator had my full support and trust. I told them repeatedly that I struggled with subtlety and needed direct communication. I thought my questions were reasonable and logical given the situation and my position, and it did not occur to me (then) that they might experience those questions differently.

Given enough time I can figure out social cues, even those that make no sense to me.

There is a pretty big time lag, though.

One of the traits characteristic of autism is a spiky cognitive profile. Allistic (nonautistic) people tend to exhibit their cognitive strengths and weaknesses within a fairly narrow range. One of the commonalities for autistic people is that our skills gaps are wider and less predictable. (This is also one of the reasons why autistic people are so very different even from each other.) I am quite brilliant given time and space to process information, but my processing speed when my nervous system is dysregulated lags by hours, days, or even weeks, and in the moment my thinking can be overly simplistic. When I do not understand what is happening, I become very dysregulated.

In retrospect I suspect that my constant questioning was creating tension long before I became aware of it. At the time I was in problemsolving mode and did what I always do when a social interaction confuses me: I asked for advice. I went to my assigned faculty mentor and asked them for help navigating the situation. I took notes on their suggestions. I started taking minutes in my meetings with the administrator so I could keep track of what was going on and verify that we were on the same page. They seemed really upset by the minutes, but I did not understand why. I was trying to be a good communicator.

The situation quickly deteriorated from there. I kept trying to problem-solve, pulling my advisers in because I could not understand where everything was going wrong. At first I was frustrated. And then I was scared. And later I felt so small and ashamed.

My body betrays me in conflict situations. It shuts down. Sometimes, if I have yet to fully process that it is a conflict situation, I keep talking. Because I have an incomplete understanding of the dynamics in play, I usually make things exponentially worse. Once I do understand an interaction as a conflict situation, I become mute. It starts with increasing curtness, and then I just cannot say anything. Until diagnosis, I never understood why. It is not my personality at all.

And because it is not my personality, others often project into my silence. They do not see the terror of being unable to control your own body, to do the things you know a leader does. They see contempt, disrespect, power plays. It never seems to occur to them that I have no control over it. The fact that I sometimes keep on talking obliviously right up until the situational mutism kicks in does not help matters.

Assumptions often become the biggest barrier for me in a work or social setting. Both science and culture normalize general-to-specific neural processing, imposing cause-and-effect narratives on individual behavior that will rarely if ever be entirely accurate for anyone and that become tangible barriers for those of us whose brains function fundamentally differently.

What fascinates me is how often these narratives serve ideology rather than humanity. For example, I know of no one, neurodivergent or not, who can keep up with the amount of email that has become the norm for faculty and administrators. And yet there is an expectation that you will reply within 24–48 hours. As long as you say you have this policy, it matters little if you actually do it. But if you say you cannot hold to it and implement boundaries, you are violating a professional norm and being difficult.

Other assumptions I came up against included seeing questions as a challenge to authority, resisting direct communication, assigning meanings and intentions to my body language or behavior, viewing sensory needs as the exclusive purview of students, and framing formal systems as a threat to community.

Consequences

My program was new, and we had yet to figure out how to meet our incredibly diverse student body's needs. Content was too fast or too slow. Assignments were too hard for some and too easy for others. Financial aid was not coming through on time or in the right amounts. Students were getting frustrated. Staff were frustrated. There were a lot of complaints.

One student kept emailing different groups of people in the administration attacking my character, chastising me for my "unprofessional[ism]" and stating I was "indifferent" and "inflexible." No one seemed to be taking the student seriously, but neither did the student face any consequences for their ad hominem attacks. I was so confused. One of us was clearly doing something wrong—either I was discriminating against the student or the student was attempting to intimidate me into giving them a grade they had not earned. Or both. But every time the student raised a fuss, the SLAC administration thanked them for sharing their thoughts and did nothing.

I knew I was supposed to somehow take charge of the situation and dissipate the tension, but I could not figure out how. I habitually use my intellect to work around moments when my body refuses to do what I want it to. But in confrontations I cannot bring my intellect to bear. I freeze.

As the student became increasingly antagonistic in class, I had no witty put-you-in-your place retort to take back command of the classroom in a way that alleviated tension and got everyone back on the same page. The best I could manage was polite, firm, and brief. I was barely able to keep speaking.

I knew the toxicity of a few students was affecting the entire program. With no idea of how to handle it, I found peer-reviewed studies on contra-power harassment that described an emerging trend of students bullying teachers. I sent the articles to my advisory committee. They said the center for teaching and learning should do some kind of presentation on the phenomenon.

I was on my own.

*　　*　　*

I trace these difficulties and their escalation to a general resistance to formal systems within the SLAC. I had already gone through the faculty hiring process and started the job before anyone got around to asking me to fill out a formal application and authorize a background check. I was hired before the governance of my position was determined in the faculty handbook and as such had no place in the organizational chart, no protections for the verbal agreements in place at my hiring, and no clear reporting line. When I asked for mediation with the administrator who became my boss, the dean handled it, but no one ever followed up to see if the issues were resolved.

Similarly, when students complained about me to the administrator with whom I had difficulties, they were thanked for sharing, but the accusations were never taken seriously. This inaction simultaneously affirmed that true accusations of discrimination would not be investigated and that false accusations could be made without consequence. These dynamics served no one.

A few months after the pandemic hit and everything went remote, the lease on my home came up for renewal. My mother was struggling, I missed my nieces, and I was miserable at my current location. I moved from Atlanta to Ohio to be closer to my family. If I liked it, I would stay and look for a job there. If I did not, I would go back when the pandemic ended and try to make it through to another academic hiring season.

I began consulting for a local nonprofit start-up almost immediately. I had clearance from my dean to do so. When I told the start-up I was ready to look for a full-time job in Ohio, they asked me to write up my own job description. My next career step solidified quickly. I grieved about leaving academia for a second time, but I could not make myself stay at the SLAC any longer.

The week I accepted this other job, I was called to meet with the dean and my boss. No one told me what the meeting was about. When I arrived I discovered another student had complained, and the dean wanted me to meet with the new chief diversity officer (CDO). I was confused, as there was an ample paper trail about the student in question, and the attacks had again been ad hominem rather than documenting specific incidents. This was a change in the organizational pattern. After the initial meeting, I asked my boss if I was being investigated. She said yes. I decided to wait to give my notice until the investigation was completed.

When I met with the CDO, I learned that my boss had passed on every complaint she had ever received about me over the years, including anonymous ones that I had never heard before. I explained my perspective and asked if anyone wanted to see the relevant documentation, as I had plenty of it. The CDO told me I was not being investigated. Beyond that, no one followed up. I was anxious to give my notice in a way that would avoid causing hardship to my students and colleagues, so I asked again if anyone wanted to see my documentation. No one did.

At first, I wondered why none of these complaints had ever been taken seriously or addressed when they occurred. That was unfair to the students and myself. Was I being investigated or not? Then a former colleague clued me in: A student had attacked me on one of the SLAC's private social media groups. That is what had directly preceded the meetings, but no one at the college had thought to tell me about it.

Finally, things made sense. They had been evaluating liability, not checking to see whether discrimination had actually occurred.

I gave my notice and was invited to speak to HR about my concerns. Based on the organization's patterns, I determined that doing so would be a waste of time.

A Change of Place

I left my faculty-administrator role in the middle of the academic year with less than two months' notice. I took another leadership role 500 miles away in an educational start-up focused on grades K–12.

Transitions, as it turned out, are very hard for me but not insurmountable. Despite changing careers and locations in the middle of a global pandemic, I was able to thrive in my new role. Nearly three years in, I am the happiest I have ever been in my professional life. I get to teach, develop curriculum, and mentor. My colleague and I took positive psychology classes together in my first year in order to incorporate the science of character strengths and resilience into our work.

Living closer to my nieces, both of whom have ADHD diagnoses, was a wake-up call regarding my own neurology. We were more alike than not.

I had a male family member who had been diagnosed as autistic when we were children. I had wondered about my differences before, as I identified more with him than with most of my family, but when I looked at the criteria, developed for white middle-class boys, I did not feel like

I quite fit. I was just really smart like my grandmother. (Fun fact: She did not speak until she was five.) It was not until I read a novel by an autistic woman about an autistic woman that I saw myself.

I did a deep dive into autistic self-advocates' perspectives. Over the next weeks, I wrote 37 pages relating my experiences to *Diagnostic and Statistical Manual V* criteria for ASD. I consulted with my therapist to get her opinion of my self-diagnosis. She agreed with my assessment.

I had to adjust everything I thought I knew about myself, but for the first time, the patterns of my own life, including why everything had gone so wrong at the SLAC, made sense.

When I pursued and received my formal diagnosis, my boss immediately asked me: How can I use this knowledge to better support you? I told her to continue doing what she had been doing—communicating directly, giving me a few moments to wrap my brain around a pivot point, and respecting my need for a narrative throughline. The glad reality was that she had already made all the accommodations I had requested. She had not needed a diagnosis in order to respect my needs.

She came up with one other very useful accommodation on her own. Knowing that I struggle with subtext in interpersonal interactions, she made sure to follow up with me after meetings with external partners to make sure I understood what went unsaid. I am cognitively capable of understanding subtext. I can identify it just fine in stories—movies or books where the audience's attention is directed to what is important. I just miss things in real life due to sensory overload and cannot interpret body language reliably as a result. These small two- or three-minute follow-ups transformed my ability to support our team and our partnerships and ensured we were on the same page as we moved forward.

With her support, I disclosed my areas of neurodivergence in my email signature line and invited parents to talk to me about it and ask me questions about how we could better support their kids. I talked to our students about it. The joy on a 10-year-old's face when I tell her that I am autistic, too, is a gift I would not change for anything.

Having had this professional experience immediately after the previous one helped me understand the structural issues that had made my previous role so toxic. From this place of understanding, support, and joy, I would like to share what I have learned about supporting neuro-divergent faculty, staff, and students.

Recommendations

Respect boundaries. Accommodate the unique communication needs of each individual. If email is hard for them, let them encourage students to use office hours. If in-person is difficult, let them use email.

People who experience delayed processing may not know what they think or feel about an interaction right away. Ways to support delayed processing include giving people important information at least 24 hours before they have the opportunity to ask questions or raise concerns. If the matter is urgent, give them the information and then allow them to take a break to process in the way that works best for them. For me, it is reducing auditory and visual input and increasing proprioceptive sensory input by rocking, walking, or otherwise moving. Conversely, one of my autistic friends needs to increase auditory input by playing music. Many of us require sensory input or avoidance in order to think.

Educate yourself about sensory differences. As one autistic professor writes, "My classroom is incredibly noisy—if you're me. Besides the constant buzz of the fluorescent lights, every computer in my room hums, as does the projector. It is so distracting that I turn all of it off when I do not have students. But it is still distracting when I have a class in session, and teaching while trying to ignore the noise can be exhausting" (Shea and Derry 2019).

Respect self-diagnosis. Within the autistic community, self-diagnosis is considered valid. The process is not usually covered by insurance. Diagnosis for adults with above-average intelligence and lower visible support needs is expensive, inefficient, and dehumanizing. For example, the clinician who formally diagnosed me still used the r-word in his paperwork.

Believe people when they tell you what they need. The professor who responds late to email or asks why all the time may be doing those things because they have to. I asked my boss at the SLAC over and over again to please communicate directly, but no matter how many times I told them I did not understand subtlety, they continued to interpret my boundaries and confusion as manifestations of ego, and as one writer notes, "When relationships do go wrong for autistic people, they can go very wrong."

Implement evidence-based workplace practices. Standardize what can be standardized. Develop policies around late papers and create grading rubrics as a department. Build a culture of trust and respect. Treat all community members' concerns seriously. Hold people accountable for the impact of their actions regardless of their intentions. Call each other in rather than out.

Conclusion

Trauma takes time to heal, and I experienced my time working at the SLAC as traumatic. Add in a global pandemic, moving, changing careers, and getting a couple of paradigm-shifting diagnoses and, well, it took me a while to decide what I wanted to do with all my new self-knowledge.

As of late 2023, I am still with the nonprofit start-up, and I love the work we do with kids. Earlier this year, I cofounded the Autistic Self-Reliance Support Network, a nonprofit focused on filling a gap in services and cultivating well-being for autistic adults. Eight months after that, my cofounder and I started a tech company to develop assistive technology for autistic people. Oh, and I also just got licensed to be a foster parent.

My plate is full. My life is full of shifts and pivots and juggling—none of which are my strengths—but I am surrounded by support.

I am open about my diagnoses. I ask for help.

And I thrive.

SEVEN

"It's All Too Much"

Finding a Place with Autism

ROBERT PERRET

I GREW UP IN A TIME before social networks: no TikTok, Facebook, or Twitter (now known as X). Not even MySpace, Friendster, or Tumblr. Our social network was the nearest convenience store that you could ride to on your bike. Our news feed was the parking lot outside where kids loitered, our comment section the bathroom stalls. This was the first social network that I was unable to navigate, but it would not be the last.

Today "social network" can mean two different things, both an on-line website where people interact with each other and, in the older sense of the phrase, the invisible spider web of connections that most people make with other people. The former is supposed to be a virtual analogue of the latter. In reality, people rack up thousands of "friends" on virtual social networks, dwarfing the number of real-life connections they have fostered. When I quit Facebook after 14 years, I had 12 Facebook friends. The theory holds. For me, 12 friends was an enormous exaggeration.

I received my autism diagnosis at the age of 44. The discovery came when my son was diagnosed by the elementary school psychologist. As we left her office, she casually mentioned, "You might want to get eval-uated too." I had been labeled difficult, defiant, insubordinate, and non-compliant, but no one, including myself, had ever considered autistic.

Back in the 1980s, when I was a child who probably should have been diagnosed, the full spectrum of autism was not well understood, especially when it came to individuals like me who did not fit the stereotypical image of being nonverbal or socially isolated. I exhibited hyperverbal tendencies, made eye contact, laughed, and even had occasional friends.

I also had my idiosyncrasies, however—reading 456 *Star Wars* books in a row, constantly checking out *The Field Guide to UFOs* from the school library for three years straight (including summers), and being argumentative with teachers when rules were inconsistently enforced or when lesson content was demonstrably incorrect. As a result I was often sent to the gifted and talented room to keep me out of the teachers' hair. This cycle of being moved around without a proper fit continued throughout elementary and middle school. In high school, academic placement was based solely on math scores. Thanks to what I would later come to know as dyscalculia, I was placed on the remedial track, and no one ever looked back.

During my upbringing, underachieving was considered a moral failing for Generation X. When I excelled in a few areas but struggled significantly in others, my struggles were brushed off as a lack of determination or effort. I chose to major in journalism because I wanted to write comic books, and it was the closest available major. My parents insisted that English was not a real subject, so majoring in it was forbidden. Additionally, journalism appealed to me because characters like Peter Parker and Clark Kent were journalists, and I could even draw a comic strip for the college paper. Best of all, there were no required math courses for a journalism degree.

In college I started my journalism career by writing CD and movie reviews. I was known for my wit and cultural references, which were valued in an entertainment reviewer. I was eventually promoted to entertainment editor, but that sat well with no one. Student reporters did not think I was cool enough. (Ironically, much of what made me uncool back then is mainstream pop culture now.) Student editors thought I was difficult to work with. (This was the year swing music was big in the 1990s, and when I pushed back on yet another swing dancing cover story, I found myself elbowed out of my own Entertainment section.)

The faculty adviser was basically absent from the role, though he would later apologize for not doing anything to intervene in my ouster. After just one semester, I was replaced.

This was my first experience witnessing a disparity between the ideals preached in academia and the actual practices. While the other students claimed to be passionate about journalism, the fourth estate, and speaking truth to power, they were more interested in house parties, internal politics, and writing fluffy pieces to appease the university. Completely oblivious to this at the time, I found myself displaced and relegated to being a "contributing writer" rather than an editor or reporter. I vividly remember a defining moment when the editor in chief assigned stories with predetermined narratives, and when I called this out, I was swiftly dismissed. It was my first lesson in the stark contrast between vision and practice in academia. From then on I wrote a few opinion columns, one of which humorously criticized the unfairness of not being allowed to take a banana from the cafeteria. It was well received and considered my best work for the paper. They only accepted me as a quirky clown; someone to laugh at, but never with.

Years later I reentered academia by enrolling in library school. The local university's library program had recently regained accreditation and was offering discounted tuition to attract students. I worked on campus, moving dusty boxes around in various basements, and did an internship at the university library. It seemed that nobody even knew my name by the time I graduated.

I took up a few postgraduate temporary jobs, one involving scanning correspondence related to Buffalo Bill Cody at the American Heritage Center. I processed thousands of documents, and when I left, nobody was sure who my supervisor even was. Simultaneously, I worked on digitizing plant specimens and field notes for the Rocky Mountain Herbarium. The person who had hired me had already left before my arrival, and their replacement was surprised to discover my existence. Nobody bothered to involve me in meetings or copy me on emails. It was then that I realized I had misunderstood the purpose of temp jobs, internships, and even college itself. People who had partied their way through, doing little work and a lot of socializing, were now succeeding while I failed, on the verge of not even graduating. That was the exact opposite of everything I had ever been told. I believed we were there to do our jobs well and be rewarded accordingly, but it seemed that networking held more importance than the work at hand. I began to understand, at least conceptually, why I was repeatedly overlooked while others effortlessly made the transition to professional positions. Prized internships were handed under the table to people who had only clocked a few hours in the archives but who had "leadership qualities." High-profile projects went to people who knew how to ask for them behind closed doors. People who "gave the right impression" were chosen to present the work that others, often me, had done. There was a whole meta-level to work that I could see the ripples of while remaining oblivious to the source.

Autism in adults receives insufficient examination, and the limited research often adopts a medical model, viewing autism as a disease or disorder and focusing on its symptoms. The one aspect that has gained some attention in literature is the social isolation experienced by adult autistics. Studies indicate that anywhere from half to three-quarters of autistic adults report being affected by social isolation on a daily basis. Even before I was diagnosed or had any inkling of being autistic, I often joked that I had "anticharisma." While I was not rude, loud, or demanding, I consistently found myself alone, akin to being in the free-reading corner, where problem children are sent so as not to bother the rest of the class.

I naturally gravitated toward history and working in archives because isolation was beneficial. In the archives the chair in the corner where I was sent to read and not bother others expanded to thousands of square feet. Immersing myself in obscure facts was a job requirement. Interactions with people were scheduled or through email. The basement was as quiet as I needed it to be, and my headphones provided the necessary escape. I could even turn off the fluorescent lights and work by desk lamp or natural sunlight during certain times of the year. On paper it was an ideal fit for someone who had been nurtured to thrive alone, and I excelled in my job. In retrospect all of the elements of these jobs that I liked were exactly the sort of accommodations sought by autistics. I had unknowingly self-accommodated.

Like most academic library archives, however, my department was closely linked to the digital projects department. They would take our materials, scan them, and place them online without seeking our input or acknowledging the archives. Even worse, that meant our materials were always missing without rhyme or reason. I could spend hours looking for an item in the archives that a digital projects person had whisked away without notice. When I pointed out this issue, even diplomatically, I was labeled as difficult. They would dump thousands of scans into an online folder and call it an archive, but it was not an archive at all. Any questions about the archives from other departments were directed to them, and they would make decisions without involving me. Problems with the metadata around items I had nothing to do with digitizing were placed back on me because describing the items was meant to be a responsibility of the archivist. They received promotions, while I failed to meet expectations. When I sought more specific feedback, I was told I needed to do more. Pressing for details only led to promises of follow-up that were never fulfilled, and once again, I failed to meet expectations.

Despite being part of a large university bureaucracy, I was evaluated by a single individual without any checks and balances or peer reviews. My request to have my reviews audited was deemed impossible. I disclosed my autism and requested informal accommodations in a meeting with my boss (trying to avoid unnecessary antagonism). The accommodations were agreed upon and even documented in an email. This only worsened the situation. The accommodations were rarely and begrudgingly honored, and I faced harsher criticism than before. Additionally, I was patronized and excluded from the few library-wide activities in which I had been previously included.

When the university ombuds came to give a presentation in the library, I learned that the office could help in cases of organizational difficulties. I scheduled a meeting with the ombuds, but he explained that his only tool was mediation and that my boss was unlikely to change. I then turned to Human Resources to have my accommodations formalized. The process took six months, and I had to continuously follow up with them for progress updates. Each time it seemed like it was the first time I had contacted them.

As a last resort, I approached the Office of Human Rights and Investigations, providing documentation of years of organizational behavior that involved ostracization, exclusion, marginalization, and, arguably, bullying. Weeks later they responded that they could only investigate a small element of my complaint unless I could demonstrate material harm.

I had followed the appropriate channels, starting small and nonconfrontational before escalating, but I finally reached a point where I had exhausted all options and received no help.

Shortly after disclosing my autism diagnosis and before losing all hope, I pursued another approach. The university had recently established a process for creating identity groups for faculty, which was pioneered by the newly formed Black Faculty Group. They created these affinity groups in response to the lack of support systems for diverse employees, despite the availability of such systems for diverse students. Recognizing that support systems for diverse people like me were unlikely to be provided, these affinity groups offered a means of self-support. I saw an opportunity and thought that by forming an autism identity group, autistic employees on campus could engage in more generalized advocacy. We could raise awareness about the needs of autistic employees and demonstrate their presence in every department and building on campus. It is easier to advocate for others and address the organization as a whole rather than individual managers who might become defensive.

I put out a call for anyone interested in starting an autism identity group, and a few people expressed interest, which met the requirement to officially establish the group. I proposed meeting times, but no one could attend. I suggested other times, but still, no one could make it. I went through the process of creating a university Teams group, but only one other person used it, and even then, only for a couple of days. Once again, I found myself alone.

The only changes I have managed to effect are internal. Through watching numerous TED Talks and reading countless articles, both popular and scholarly, I now understand myself better. I comprehend my limitations and how they compare to the neurotypical experience. I can set reasonable goals for myself and engage in appropriate self-care without feeling guilty. For example, I block out time for decompression after meetings or limit the number of obligations I take on in a day. I even use a chatbot to soften the tone of my emails before sending them. I am better able to interpret the harsh tone of others (the double empathy problem is a real challenge) and assign their criticisms to myself, to autism, or to their neurotypical 24/7 grind culture, as appropriate. I am human so I accept responsibility for some things, but I am autistic, and some things are not my fault. I have never subscribed to the 24/7 grind mentality that seems to be expected of everyone, including librarians.

I also volunteer for every diversity, equity, and inclusion (DEI) group that emerges. Unfortunately, neurodiversity is rarely considered by these groups. Neurodiverse conditions are either viewed as symptoms of more obvious disabilities or labeled as "superpowers." Since becoming a public advocate for neurodiverse people in academia, I have experienced both reactions.

As a result, opportunities to lead or chair groups or projects unrelated to DEI have vanished. I am no longer assigned to hiring committees, and within my library, I am barely given any projects at all. There is now a perception that I cannot be trusted with significant responsibilities. Any delay, hiccup, or missed target is attributed to my autism. The natural irregularities of work not even worth mentioning when they happen to my peers are framed as insurmountable obstacles that I have created for myself. On the other hand, when I publish a book, it is hardly acknowledged because it is assumed that I can effortlessly produce manuscripts. I am seen either as a superhuman savant or a bumbling fool with malicious intent. As long as I am considered the problem, as I have always been told, these perceptions persist.

I see my son being confined to the same boxes in school. That is why I proudly wear an autism acceptance pin and openly identify as autistic in meetings, conferences, and even when teaching classes. Despite the recent emphasis on DEI, autistic individuals and other diverse people who do not quite fit in continue to be ostracized and diminished. The Centers for Disease Control and Prevention reports that 2.8% of eight-year-olds are diagnosed with autism, and that statistic does not even account for older individuals. Autism often goes undiagnosed until later, particularly among women and individuals who are Black, Indigenous, or people of color. The minimum estimate is 2.8%, meaning it equates to 1 in 36 people. Statistically, most public schools would have at least 1 autistic student per classroom, yet very few supports are in place for these students. At the undergraduate level, there would be several autistic students in large courses. Do professors ever consider how to support autistic students? Do colleges ever consider how to support autistic faculty?

Being diagnosed later in life means being born into a strange and incomprehensible culture. It involves living a cursed life, facing insurmountable personal challenges, and experiencing inexplicable hostility from a world that treats everyone else more kindly. Naming the curse does not remove it, but it does reveal its dimensions. I now wonder what my life would have been like if I had been diagnosed as a child. How would I be different today? Would I be happier but less successful in my career? Would I have faced further marginalization by being placed in alternative programs outside the mainstream academic tracks? In those days accommodations for students facing nontrivial learning challenges were not additional support programs, or classroom aides, or extra testing time. It was banishing those students to a vestigial world of life skills classes and job training programs, or worse. The question was not how to lift them up, but how to get them out of the way.

The fight to fit into a world that rejects me has exhausted me. It is a battle to keep up with individuals who are better suited for this environment while I struggle to breathe in an atmosphere that fails to cater to my needs. I did not deserve this and neither does my son. As a result, I no longer find myself alone in the silent-reading corner; instead, I am present at the table, raising my voice in the silences. I hold the academic institutions I am part of accountable for their commitment to diversity, equity, and inclusion. My divergent brain affects everything I do, and true diversity means accommodating that diversity rather than punishing it. Equity involves providing equal opportunities, support, and evaluations regardless of personal likability. Inclusion means being remembered and involved when decisions are made and groups are formed. It means having the same stake in the organization as any other faculty member. It means being spoken with, not spoken about. I am now aware of myself, academia, and the hidden elements that were once concealed from me. I cannot rewrite my own history, but I can rewrite the history my son will experience, just as he has rewritten mine.

I previously mentioned my exodus from the world of virtual social networks. Social media is just too much, all the time: too much content, too much vitriol, too many algorithms, too many charismatic influencers steamrolling everyone else. But that is not just social media; that is real-world social networks too. I do not like it, I do not understand it, and I am not any good at it. I will spend my whole life punished by this demonstrably artificial system of interaction. What gets clicks, and likes, and followers is not meaningful engagement with life. It is people who have "leadership qualities" and who "give the right impression" who profit, as always. And, as always, I was too slow to learn this and am unable to adapt.

Just as I left social media, I have now left academia. I tried for years to make the situation better, through the ombuds office, Human Resources, and even the Office for Civil Rights. I did everything I was supposed to do, again, and it was turned against me, again. After 15 years I have finally learned that I cannot benefit from the system, navigate the system, or even coexist with the system. I certainly cannot beat the system. In the end my only avenue of appeal to the social network of academia was to unfollow.

EIGHT

Both Can Be True

Risk and Protective Factors for Bipolar Prognosis in Academia

DARCY GORDON

AT FIRST, I THOUGHT this message was spam: "Dear Dr. Gordon, Hope you are doing well. [Our department] at MIT is leading a diversity and inclusion effort. As a part of the initiative, we invite prominent research- ers around the world to talk about their research and their journey to become a successful researcher. It is our great pleasure to invite you to give a 50 mins presentation." I had just transitioned out of my postdoc- toral position and was newly appointed as an instructor of blended and online learning in the Department of Biology at MIT (Massachusetts Institute of Technology). In this role I help make teaching more effective with technology and collaborate with faculty to develop and maintain Massive Open Online Courses based on the subjects that the department teaches. I am well accustomed to creatively addressing academic chal- lenges in my discipline but not exactly a "prominent researcher," at least, not on the scale of MIT. When I realized this message was sincere, a surging wave of appreciation quickly crashed into doubt. The format of the talk was part diversity, equity, and inclusion (DEI) seminar, part per- sonal reflection, and part research talk. I was tasked with speaking to something deeply personal, in addition to my subject-matter expertise.

When talking to my wife later, I was not sure how to approach this request. As a queer, white woman with bipolar disorder who has been in educational systems from kindergarten through a PhD, I had difficulty teasing apart these facets of my identity within academia. How could I make sense of it all? She, a public health professional in the field of violence prevention, remarked that this dilemma was something she often confronts in her work. She uses a socioecological approach to describe how risk and protective factors are nested within individual, interpersonal, community, and societal levels (Golden and Earp 2012). Like some meta-matryoshka doll, the model describes how these nested layers influence our health outcomes. Factors at the individual level include biological and social history. The interpersonal level is composed of close relationships that influence behavior and mindset, which are situated within a broader community (in the case of higher education, this is the university or institution) that has its own structure and characteristics that provide context for the interpersonal interactions. All these factors are further couched within a society that operates with specific social and cultural norms.

Ideas started to click into place. As I reflected on my whiteness, womanhood, and queerness, I started to understand how my mental health disability was affected not only by these other parts of myself but by the relationships, institutional supports, and cultural norms within academia. By applying this socioecological model to my own story, I could have a better understanding of how my bipolar disorder and other identities shape my experiences in higher education. Throughout my schooling, I felt erasure and exclusion, as well as respite and refuge. Even though now I am a staff member at an elite R1 institution and years removed from formal schooling, I still carry the positive and negative experiences throughout my education with me in my current role. The nuanced social and cultural factors that influenced these experiences remain relevant in today's academic landscape. By telling my story in this socioecological framework, I am able to articulate the need for radical vulnerability and authenticity within the academy throughout these nested levels of organization. I believe that by answering this call, we can cocreate environments rich in empathy, connection, and mutual respect so that all students, faculty, and staff members can thrive.

Individual Factors, White Privilege, and Mental Health Care

I was on a path to higher education well before I ever stepped foot on a college campus. We know that childhood experiences, like high school math coursework, affect the likelihood of earning a postsecondary degree (Tyson et al. 2007). So we enter this story in early high school at the time of my bipolar symptom onset. Sleepless nights gave way to frenzied work on dramatic interpretations of academic assignments. When I needed to recite a monologue in literature class, "All the World's a Stage" was my choice. In art class I needed to interpret a societal problem, and I chose depression and suicide to decorate my page. AP American history was punctuated by the occasional outburst fueled by surging emotions and the whispers of clueless peers. Later the tranquilizers, antipsychotics, and mood stabilizers would slow my typically pressured speech in poetry class to an exaggerated drawl. Throughout these disruptions, my teachers would simply send me to the nurse to cool down, cry it out, or sometimes take a nap. And despite all that volatility, I still wore the cords of a valedictorian as I accepted my diploma.

Looking back, my racial identity likely buffered me against some of the most severe consequences for a volatile teen in a high school community. Teachers, like everyone else, harbor racial biases (Starck et al. 2020), and we know that across U.S. public schools, the disciplinary consequences for Black girls is greater than those of their white peers (Hill 2018). The perception of teachers was not the only way in which my identities influenced my treatment. Anyone who needs behavioral health interventions should have access to them. And yet racial disparities in mental health care are well-documented. Extending beyond the time I was finishing high school (Cook et al. 2017) and more recently during the COVID-19 pandemic (Thomeer et al. 2023), mental health care systems fail to meet the needs of Black, Asian, and Hispanic individuals compared to their white peers.

So a confluence of individual factors like my positionality, family dynamics, and geographic location meant that I was under the care of professionals and monitored by adults who cared about me. These protective qualities and relationships helped offset my painful adolescence and ensured I had access to the care that I needed. Many of the attributes encompassed within the individual level of the socioecological model, however, are not within our control. We can be honest with our needs and find the courage to ask for help, but that is only a first step. Robust mental health care requires the coordination of multiple systems, and the people operating within them, to consistently and equitably offer treatment options.

Interpersonal Factors, Substance Abuse, and Gendered Violence

Emboldened by my newfound adult freedom on my college campus, I decided to be proactive. I made an appointment with my university's counseling service almost immediately. After a couple of sessions, I was told they did not have the capacity to treat such chronic cases as my own. With well-wishes and a half-hearted suggestion to seek out private care, I was dismissed. After a year or so, my symptoms got worse. Insomnia, hypomania, and suicidal ideation continued to plague me. I decided to take an incomplete for the semester, go home, and finish my work with extensions.

I needed a plan for completing my course requirements, so I reached out to my professors—first, my chemistry research adviser. "I'm leaving the semester early," I said. "I'm bipolar and my meds—," but midsentence, I was cut off. "Look, I don't care what goes on outside of the lab; that's your business and not mine," he interrupted. "Just leave your notebook in a shape where you can pick back up when you return." Shocked into silence, I packed up and headed to my calculus professor's office. "Tell me what's going on," she invited. "I have bipolar disorder, and my medication isn't working. I need to take an incomplete, but I'll finish up later this month," I responded. "What does it mean that the medication isn't working?" she pried further. "I'm not sleeping or I'm sleeping too much, my brain is foggy, I'm still depressed, and now I have tremors in my hands," I explained. "Oh! I feel so terrible for you! That must be so hard. That just makes me . . . so . . . sad!" she wept. "It's really ok. I'm ok," I reassured her, unconvinced. I walked away with my remaining coursework outlined and a reminder of how alone I felt.

Despite taking time at home and a new psychotropic cocktail, I felt the need to self-medicate. I thought I was taking charge of my life where other options had failed to regulate my mood. In reality, alcohol mixed with prescription medication in the body of a young woman under severe psychological distress made me extremely vulnerable. On a night like many others when I had too much to drink, I was sexually assaulted. When I tried to seek support, I was met with blame from my peers and cold bureaucracy from staff. My memory was shoddy, my affect was inconsistent, and my reputation was not exactly spotless. I was a messy victim. I cracked jokes at my own expense, desperately fishing for someone to correct me. No one did. My messiness undermined my credibility and gave others an excuse to withhold empathy when I needed it most.

Alcohol and substance use and abuse in people with bipolar disorder (Cassidy et al. 2001) and queer youth (Hoots et al. 2023) are more prevalent than in the general public. Somewhat ironically, the only time I had reliable mental health care in college was when I was mandated to attend substance-abuse counseling as a condition of my collegiate disciplinary probations. At no point during those sessions did the counselor probe meaningfully into why I felt like I needed to self-medicate. What was going on with me that made this behavior feel necessary? If someone asked, I may have told them that it made me feel alive, it cut through the pain and made me feel good about myself, and it allowed me to be in my body without feeling the crushing weight of the trauma it held. Sexual violence against college-aged women is disturbingly common (Cantor et al. 2019), especially toward those with mental health disabilities (Bonomi et al. 2018) and bisexual women of any age (Chen et al. 2020).

When reflecting back on what could have been different in my college experience and what could be different for others in the future, the most tangible points of intervention are at the interpersonal level of the socioecological model: the interactions I had with my peers, professors, and university staff. The reactions I received when I talked to others about my mental health, substance abuse, or trauma were terribly inconsistent, as illustrated before. Believing our students' and peers' experiences are real is the first step to enacting a different kind of system. Extending empathy and respect naturally comes next. I cannot say that if the people around me were kinder that these things would not have happened. I can say, though, that if my well-being was truly valued by the university and my peers, perhaps I would have valued it more myself, and I could have processed and coped with the traumas more easily.

Community Factors, Academics, and Queer Solidarity

Fortunately, I had an opportunity to change my scenery and shift my focus. I swapped oak trees for banyans and immersed myself in a summer research experience in Singapore. Although it was already late at night for my parents, my day was just beginning. The hum of the air conditioner working overtime hushed the sounds of the street vendors. "I think I have found my passion," I told them over the long-distance call. I was truly living the values of our household mantra, "Have fun and learn a lot." I was eager to know more and worked hard to get there. Over those eight weeks, I became a proficient navigator of the controls at the confocal microscope and trained my hand in dissections and DNA extractions. I looked up to my mentor and saw in her my potential future reflected back. My involvement in research sustained me throughout the semesters remaining in my undergraduate career and propelled me into a master's degree program and later a PhD.

Sensory neurobiology, phenotypic plasticity, and behavioral ecology were among my favorite graduate courses. Together they asked: How do brain anatomy, neurochemistry, and synaptic structure produce the stunning variation in behavior across all animal life? This question drew me in because I had a similar question of my own. I wanted to know: How does that chaotic mass of neurons bathed in chemicals produce my thoughts, impulses, and actions with which I so often struggle? In a way, my bipolar disorder diagnosis spurred a curiosity that I could channel into scientific inquiry. My science was driven by a deeply personal connection to neuroethology, or the neurobiological basis of behavior, as I studied how body morphology, brain anatomy, and social behavior covaried in different ant species. I also was not alone. In graduate school I was surrounded by a cohort of budding academics who were also intimately interested in their study systems and were facing similar challenges to manage their projects while also navigating young adulthood in a new city. We spoke openly about our mental health and personal lives. Rainbow flags and festive banners decorated the office year-round, not just for Pride in June. There was a sense of safety (both emotional and physical) in our little corner of the Biology Research Building.

Every day the ants in the lab went about their tasks, foraging on routes and caring for larvae. On a November morning in 2016, they proceeded as usual in their standardized artificial habitats. We, too, tended to our scientific and teaching duties, as expected, but found ourselves in a changed political landscape. Observing their tiny world normally brought me calm and wonder; however, I now found myself feeling helpless and small. The day dragged on, my eyes puffy and unfocused staring blankly at my computer screen, cheeks stained with mascara. A gentle knock on the office door brought me back into my body. Slightly slouched in the doorway stood the only openly queer professor in our program. "I wanted to check in with this office today," she said. Soon a chorus of questions interrupted the previously solemn silence. "What does this mean for my health care?" "My partner is not a citizen—how will this affect immigration?" "Will it be safe to travel to other states?" The underlying subtext was "What will happen to us?" Although there were no answers given, that pause to acknowledge our shared reality, by a person in power no less, helped bolster our spirits and reaffirmed our connections to each other.

The fact that many of my peers similarly struggled with anxiety and depression was not a fluke. Approximately 40% of graduate students in the United States report suffering from clinical symptoms of anxiety or depression (Evans et al. 2018). Queer representation in STEM is also lacking, and hostile environments push out talented queer scientists (Cech and Waidzunas 2021). Perhaps it is no surprise that we see a mental illness epidemic among graduate students (queer and otherwise identified). They are tasked with the daunting feat of generating new knowledge, often have their identities intertwined with their academic success, and are put into a high-stress environment that endures for years. I would also argue that academia attracts bright people who may already struggle with mental health. What other industry rewards individuals for obsessive rumination and offers loosely defined timelines for deliverables? This is all the more reason why universities should invest energy and resources into social supports for students and staff alike. One kind professor or staff member who wants to check in with their students is not enough to sustain an inclusive academic ecosystem.

Formalized institutional supports could help build community, distribute responsibility to prevent burnout, and increase workplace satisfaction. At MIT these kinds of social supports manifest as funding student organizations, hiring departmental DEI officers, and offering employee resource groups (ERGs). I am a part of both the QStaff (LGBTQIA+ identified staff members) and Disabilities ERGs. The community fostered by these groups is empowering, as cross-membership helps identify inclusive, intersectional approaches to improving the staff experience from multiple angles. These are excellent initiatives, and they are necessary but not sufficient for maintaining supportive spaces. These programs and positions not only need ongoing financial and administrative investment but an environment in which their work is amplified, uplifted, and seen as vital infrastructure to a healthy university.

Societal Factors and Coming Out Mentally Ill

I admit that I masked my mental health disability when I first arrived at MIT. I was thrown into a panic when I filled out the application for my earlier postdoctoral associate position. It was close to the review deadline, and I was copying and pasting the details of my curriculum vitae into the online forms. Thinking I had completed the task, I was caught completely off guard by that simple checkbox asking if I would like to disclose a disability. I was so afraid that this would jeopardize my chances (despite legal protections), and I questioned how this information would be used. I could hear the thuds of my quickening heartbeat against my temples as I clicked "Decline to answer." Only after my first few years of work did I tell my supervisor about my mental health. And it was not until after I was promoted to my role as instructor that I formally disclosed my disability status to Human Resources.

I still struggle with a combination of internalized ableism and realistic appraisal of the ongoing stigma associated with bipolar disorder that American society perpetuates. Otherwise well-meaning colleagues describe unexpected interactions as "crazy," wise-cracking peers as "nuts," and many make jokes about addiction. These subtle signals make me feel like I cannot truly be open with my diagnoses and experiences. Moreover, I work in an environment steeped in the traditions of science, where the myth of objectivity still reigns. When having hard conversations with coworkers, my face gets hot and my throat tightens, sure signs that tears are on the horizon, so I try to drink water to ground myself and take a pause. To protect my professionalism, I actively stifle my emotions and employ all the skills I have to regulate my affect. As a demonstrative and labile person, this is not an easy task. This struggle between authenticity and credibility was brought into focus with the speaker invitation that began this retrospective reflective process. How could I talk about my academic journey without mentioning the prominent role my mental health played throughout my experiences?

Ultimately, I accepted the invitation and prepared my talk. I wanted to be part of the movement at MIT to make disability a more visible part of the conversation about DEI. I was pleased that they were investing in these seminar series, and I wanted to do my part in demonstrating that there is both supply and demand for disabled stories at the institute. When the time came, I logged onto the Zoom meeting, shared my screen, and began talking to the dozens of attendees that joined but whom I could not see. It was a surreal experience. In one sense I felt anonymous; it was just me talking alone in my apartment to my computer screen. And yet I was also intimately vulnerable. I "came out" with my mental illness disability and described how this interfaced with each stage of my educational experience and other identities.

At the end of the seminar, I felt immense pride and relief. Soon after I received several emails thanking me for speaking candidly about mental illness. One faculty member said, "[You] discussed and modeled important issues for this community . . . such an integrated statement is extremely rare. . . . [You] did a service, both to this place and to many individuals whom you lifted up." And one from a graduate student included, "This is the first time I have ever heard anyone in the biology department openly talk about their mental illness. . . . I am glad that there is someone as open and authentic as you in our department to help remove the stigma of having a mental illness." It was validating to hear that by telling my story, I could help others feel less alone or more aware.

I believe that authenticity, or adhering to our values in words and actions, is critical to forging more transparent and fulfilling relationships. Practicing radical vulnerability (e.g., Sjunneson 2020) means that we do not hide our true feelings nor do we carelessly blurt out the details of our innermost thoughts. We purposefully share our experiences and emotional reactions, leading with compassion for ourselves and others. Authenticity coupled with radical vulnerability enables us to courageously make our intentions known, act in accordance with what we know about ourselves, and invite others to know us deeply. In doing so, we build connections that counteract the isolation pervading many of our shared spaces.

Radical Vulnerability and Authenticity in Higher Education

What do radical vulnerability and authenticity look like in academia? At the individual level of the socioecological model, we can embrace the fact that individuals are the experts of their own lives and shift to accept our own strengths and flaws with equal attention. I try to remain accountable, take ownership for my choices, and extend compassion to myself whenever I can. This radical expression of self-knowledge may have the intended side effect of acknowledging that others have rich lives of which outsiders are mostly unaware. This can inform our interpersonal relationships. Faculty and staff would benefit from approaching interactions with students and peers with curiosity and openness. For example, avoiding the assumption that everyone has the same academic and cultural background can create opportunities that open discussion to different perspectives. Even more so, modeling our own authentic vulnerability to others encourages them to engage with their whole selves in turn. In the emails I received after my talk, folks opened up about their own mental health issues and asked questions on how to support their students and loved ones.

Creating a culture where everyone feels empowered to speak their truths and mutually respect others' will form a foundation for broader institutional efforts. Over the past several years, I developed an online inclusive teaching module and companion workshop series for the MIT community and beyond (Gordon 2022). This project has helped me transform some of the pain from my tumultuous days as an undergraduate. By helping train future and current faculty how to be more aware, empathetic, and welcoming teachers, I am able to help cocreate learning environments where everyone feels cared for and valued, something my younger self needed desperately. On a more systemic scale, universities can enact equitable policies, like hybrid working and learning. Equitable strategies collectively operate with the diversity and unpredictability of life circumstances in mind. Universities are hubs of information, incubators of innovation, and, at places like MIT, models for policy on a global stage. At multiple levels, enacting justice in education readies the next generations for a more humane future together. We must face our complicated histories and accept a more nuanced and vulnerable reality to prepare ourselves as teachers and students in that bold possibility. To that end I have chosen to believe that I am neither all my successes nor all my suffering; I am not only harmed or completely healed. I acknowledge both can be true.

NINE

Am I the Problem?

Anxiety, Ambition, and Belonging in Higher Education

REBECCA POPE-RUARK

WHEN I TOOK on my first role as a tenure-track faculty member, straight out of graduate school, I thought I was in heaven. Despite being academically ambitious, I had never fancied myself as someone cut out for a flagship R1 or an Ivy League institution. I dreamed about a beautiful liberal arts college focused on undergraduate education and growing in national recognition for innovation. That is where I landed. I had a full-time role in an English department, teaching exactly what I wanted to be teaching, at an institution that highly valued a liberal arts education and the art of pedagogy; a beautiful brick and colonnade-lined place with ambitious undergraduates and smart colleagues who cared deeply about the success of our students. I could thrive here, become a master teacher, do scholarly research that mattered, succeed, and get the attention I craved by being smart and capable and innovative.

Fast-forward 11 years. I sit in a scarcely used stairwell on campus, trying to breathe past the elephant sitting on my chest, cursing that I forgot to bring my Xanax. I am squashed under the weight of what I did today and what I will have to come back and do tomorrow and, ridiculously, what I should have for lunch. I had just spent 3 hours in a large room with 10 juniors and seniors looking at me disapprovingly, regretting their decision to participate in a semester-long design-thinking program I had spearheaded with several colleagues. For those 3 hours I tried to teach, facilitate, be positive, and stay out of their way, even though I felt the burden of their disapproval and growing indifference in my core.

The program I imagined changing higher education was not working, no matter what we/I did to pivot or adapt or prototype. Three years' worth of work and persistence and pushing and stress for something that was failing to be, in reality, what we had imagined with such excitement. And me, the one faculty member with the students every day, three hours a day, four or five days a week, failing at the only thing I ever really thought I was truly good at. It left me so unable to focus I could not even write about the program to get some research publications out of it and, therefore, make it "worth it"; so weak I could not get from the building to my car without crashing in the stairwell trying not to hyperventilate; so broken that I was practically in tears (again) over being unable to decide what to have for lunch.

How did I get here? Am I the problem? Or does the structure of higher education share the blame?

*　*　*

When I was in high school, I got out of physical education thanks to a doctor's note from my allergist. My diagnosis? Exercise-induced asthma. Every time I would get ready for gym class in junior high, changing into ill-fitting shorts and a school T-shirt in the locker room surrounded by other girls at various stages of development, I would start to feel it: something in my chest. By the time I got downstairs to the gym, the weight pressing down would get heavier. I could feel the attack coming on. And god forbid I had to actually exercise in front of the other kids, whether it be shooting hoops or playing volleyball (I am nearsighted in one eye and farsighted in the other, so anything with a ball was torture) or doing some test like seeing how many push-ups we could do while everyone else stared at you (my record was one-half). Very rarely did I not end a gym period without some level of chest pain and hyperventilation. It would sometimes take hours for my breathing to even out and my chest to expand. Hence the doctor's note.

It is easy to look back and wonder how my parents and my doctors missed what was really going on. But it was the early 1990s, and no one in my steel town was looking for panic attacks in children. I was not correctly diagnosed until graduate school, when I landed in the health center convinced I was having a heart attack in the midst of some family drama and school overwhelm. When the cardiac tests came back normal, they gave me a few Xanax and sent me home with a prescription for anxiety meds, a better understanding of the physical reactions my body was having to stress, and a rejoinder to try therapy.

It was a revelation. How many times had I ended up in the emergency room getting breathing treatments when I was overwhelmed in college or worried about a relationship? These treatments never worked, though no doctor ever seemed to notice. How many times had I gotten out of something at school or home that made me, what I would now call, severely anxious because of my "asthma" attacks? Or what about the childhood fixations about our house catching fire or the bump on my wrist I was sure was cancer?

So much in my young life to that point finally made sense. I had a panic disorder and generalized anxiety disorder as well as depression, and it was directly tied to my need to succeed in academics. Why did gym class in particular give me panic attacks? Because I was bad at anything that required physical movement and hand-eye coordination, even with glasses and bifocals. I regularly got hit in the face with a volleyball, could not judge the distance to the basketball hoop, and was generally clumsy and uncoordinated. And as someone who learned that her place in the family and social hierarchy was as "the smart one," being bad at anything at school was unthinkable, let alone being so bad so publicly. It went against my entire identity and the sense that school was where I belonged and where I could fit in. I was ashamed to be bad at something. So I panicked every single time. Anything that threatened that view of myself and school was to be avoided or subverted. So that is what I did (or did not do, depending on how you look at it).

My intelligence was my identity growing up, the thing that got me positive attention and made me special. My younger sister had a chronic illness that kept my mother focused on her care, so I got attention through academic success. I was the type of kid who was born (or made, I guess) for higher education, both as a student and a faculty member. Bira and Evans (2019) note that "rigorous training programs select top-tier students who have much of their identity tied up in high performance and achievement. Such identity is greatly challenged during the course of training and into the career span; the demands of academia consistently confront individuals with their own shortcomings, promote unrealistic upward social comparisons, and drive high standards of approval. This easily sets the stage for symptoms of burnout, anxiety, and depression, particularly for those with other known vulnerability factors."

As you will see, this was definitely me. In a way, higher education is a trap for neurodiverse faculty (and staff and students). We were socialized to conceal or bury anything that smacks of an "unhealthy" mind and to shame ourselves if our brains are not functioning in a neurotypical and rational way (Hoban and Hesson 2021, 39).

*   *   *

I tried the "real world" for a couple of years between my master of arts and PhD programs. I moved to California to work at a marketing communications firm in Silicon Valley, far away from everyone I knew. If I learned anything from that job, it was that my place was in academia. I was not meant for nine to five, shilling servers and now-obsolete digital devices. I did not understand how to write for sales or what the products did or even how to find out. I was depressed, lonely, and having panic attacks on the way to the office for most of my time there. When I quit after less than 18 months, I was on probation with my boss, who said I was not meeting the needs of our clients and was costing them money with my slow writing. Because I was in shock when he told me I had a month to meet a page-long list of criteria he had created, I did not tell him how much my clients told me they liked what I was producing, despite his red-pen murder of my copy. So, two weeks after the probation meeting, I called my own meeting, saying I quit and wanted to go back to school for my PhD. It was a fib at the time; I had nowhere to go. I just could not imagine being in a place where I was a failure any longer. It went against my identity as the smart one.

But I did return to the place where I felt safe—academia. I managed to get into the PhD program of my choice just a few weeks before the semester started, so I assumed it was destined to be. I would be a college professor. I would read, discuss, and write. I would always be learning. I would teach, and enlighten, and prepare students for the future. I would belong and be happy.

It did not take too long before this romanticized notion of higher ed started to crack under the weight of stress and my anxiety. I needed a 4.0 grade point average to reaffirm my belonging every semester. I needed people to see that I was smart and capable and worthy of my place in the program. The panic attacks began again in earnest pretty quickly after I started the program. My first semester, I took two electives tangentially related to my major because I had registered for classes so late. Neither were particularly relevant to my intellectual interests, so I had difficulty engaging and enjoying learning. I found myself crying regularly to my then-fiancé, and I am not a crier. From my bedroom in a shared house with other students, I would do my homework, anxiety always just below the surface. What if I did not belong here? What if I hated all my classes as much as these two? Where was I supposed to go?

Also that semester, I taught two sections of undergraduate business communication in the late afternoon. I thought I was doing a good job. I had won a teaching award during my master's program, after all. But when I read my course evaluations from that semester, I sank into a major panic attack, convinced the program director was going to kick me out of school for being a terrible teacher. Several, but not all, of the students eviscerated me. They attacked my teaching, my personality, my patterns of speech. The director called me into her office. I spent the hour before sweating, my heart pounding, my ears ringing, and my chest tight but carefully planning what I would say and do in the meeting when she fired me so I did not out myself as "too emotional." The director was actually wonderful and helped me understand how to read the evaluations critically, how to find the nuggets of feedback that would actually help me improve my teaching, and how to let the rest roll off my back (she recommended reading with a healthy glass of wine).

Then, in my third year, I actually quit my program. Well, kinda. At the time I was finishing my coursework and ready to move into my comp exam and dissertation phase. I had chosen a dissertation topic and adviser based on a seminar paper I had written that seemed to have the most legs. I spent a lot of hours that year in panic mode. Even though I thought academia was the only place I could belong, to that point in time I had never truly believed I would have anything new to say or contribute to empirical research in my field, or any field. And as courses wrapped up, I panicked that that would be when they realized I was a fraud, had nothing new to say, and did not belong in the program. I had panic attacks when my adviser did not return my emails immediately; when I thought for longer than a couple of minutes about the topic I had chosen; when I realized that the project would take more years of research than I wanted to commit to being a PhD student. I experienced lots of panic attacks, popping Xanax like candy.

One ordinary day on my 30-minute drive to campus, the panic receded, and my mind became clear. I had to quit. I could not keep living like this. I felt preternaturally calm for the first time in years. I remember thinking that the absence of panic must mean this is the right decision. So I got to campus and went to my first meeting with my Preparing Future Faculty Program adviser and told her I quit. She looked a little stunned and suggested I talk to our department's assistant chair. I showed up in his office—he a gruff, baseball-loving, lovable old-timer—and proceeded to weep. It all tumbled out: my anxiety about my adviser and my topic, my imposter syndrome, my panic attacks. He also looked stunned, told me it would be all right, and then suggested I talk to the professor next door (who was a woman). I think my weeping freaked him out.

I did talk to the professor next door, the woman who would become my dissertation adviser and get me out the door in two years. As I cried, she told me nothing was set in stone, that I had time to decide, that I needed to go home and get some rest, and that we would discuss my future in the program tomorrow or next week. I went home and slept for most of the day as the panic hangover wore off. The next morning, in the shower, I came up with the idea that would ultimately be my dissertation. This pattern of stressing out about an idea or paper or article and having a full-blown panic meltdown followed by a brilliant rush of productivity would haunt me for years to come.

*　　*　　*

By my count, this experience in my third year of the PhD was my second flirtation with burnout that dramatically exacerbated my anxiety and panic disorders. I would flirt when finishing my dissertation and then again, dramatically and decisively, 11 years into my faculty career. My episode in the stairwell at my perfect job was one of many that year. The program I had worked so hard to create and make real, that I was told could change higher education if it worked, just did not work. All that research and dreaming and scheming and work amounted to failure.

I had not just been fighting for the program, though. I had been fighting to honor my own ambition in the only place I thought I knew how to be successful. It seemed that everyone around me was taking on a leadership role, leading a center, becoming nationally known. But what about me? This program was supposed to lead to the validation I had craved since I was a child, the acknowledgment that I was worthy of not just belonging but succeeding and innovating in this academic space, this space driven by productivity, hustle, striving. This place will always demand more of you even as you give it everything you have, and because academia is a calling, not just a job, and a vocation, not just a career, we continue to give until we burn out. And I did, epically.

So am I the problem? Do my ambitions and shortcomings create conditions for so much stress, anxiety, and panic? Or is higher ed, especially the holy grail narrative of the tenure track, equally to blame? Is higher ed the perfect place for someone like me or hell? My anxiety loved the predictability of higher ed, the turnover of semesters year to year, the preset hoops to jump through for promotion, and even the constant evaluation of my work by others—more people to tell me I am worthy (or not). It seemed straightforward from the outside when I was leaving industry and fleeing to higher ed: publish, teach well, serve, and poof!—tenure. Ha!

But, eventually, you realize that whatever you can do in teaching, research, and service will never be enough, no matter how much of yourself and your well-being you give (Knights and Clarke 2014, 338; Thomason 2012, 30). Faculty participants in a study by David Knights and Caroline Clarke (2014) called academia a "treadmill" on which you have to always "be excellent" because "the job is never done; it's never done properly, and it's never done well enough. You're always feeling terribly guilty" (339–344). This level of conflict between higher ed's hustle culture and overextending expectations, on the one hand, and a need for a sense of belonging and fulfillment, on the other, contributes to burnout (Sabagh et al. 2018, 132). And that conflict creates a culture that is often isolating and competitive. Knights and Clarke (2014) summarize multiple studies, finding higher ed a place where "competitiveness, intellectualism, achievement-orientation, hierarchy, and evaluativeness [may give rise to] all manner of high emotions, anxieties, defenses, denials, deceptions and self-deceptions, rivalries, insecurities, threats, vulnerabilities, [and] intimacies" (338).

I had wrapped my entire identity, anxiety and all, around what higher ed culture told me success was—scholarly productivity, strong teaching, more service commitments than I could manage, awards, leadership appointments, and just plain and simple external recognition. It was what I craved; it was what I needed to validate who I am as a person. Without that validation I was striving to reach ideals I did not really believe in and heights I was not that interested in. Did I really want all the responsibility of leading a big program or center? Or did I just want the title because that was the next thing on the ladder on my way to full professor? When your self-worth is wrapped up in what other people define as success and that bar keeps moving, of course my anxiety ran rampant. Eventually (after two breakdowns, medical leave, therapy, and meds), I realized I was never going to be enough on the path I was on with my kind of ambition tempered with anxiety.

Vera Dolan (2023) asks, "What happens when a professor has some form of invisible differentness that, if detected, would be considered a disability and therefore a potential liability to their reputation?" (689) She refers to "invisible disability" as "a mental, cognitive, or physical impairment that is not easily detectable by an observer" (690). Higher education is grounded in the mind, the rational, and the logical, and to have an invisible disability or mental illness seems antithetical to "the profession that considers intellect to be a person's most valuable asset" (690). In summarizing the extensive literature, Housel (2023) argues that a "culture of silence historically surrounds the issue of mental illness in an academic profession where not being able to cope with the rigors of research, teaching, and service is viewed as personal weakness" (6). And Meluch (2023) notes that issues like depression and anxiety are fraught in higher education, where an academic experiencing these issues is "often perceived as incompetent, weak, and even dangerous" and as "not being able to cope with the job's daily rigors and seemingly never-ending workload" (35).

My invisible disability, severe anxiety, thrives in higher education because, as Johnson and Lester (2021) argue, "Many symptoms of mental and emotional distress among faculty can be masked by the very tendencies toward overwork and perfectionism that academia selects for, and faculty are often encouraged in this very behavior. The messages many receive from mentors and colleagues about how to manage the stress, anxiety, and pressure associated with academic life often involve some version of 'work harder,' 'focus more on productivity,' or 'be grateful for the flexibility of academia.'"

I do not know if anyone ever told me these things point blank, but I certainly picked them up through observation and osmosis. To this day, five years after that moment in the stairwell and the burnout breakdown that changed my professional life, I still struggle with thinking I am not *doing* enough or *producing* enough to be safe in higher ed. The academic culture creates pressures and conditions that "can contribute to, exacerbate, or even instigate mental health challenges for faculty and students alike" (Johnson and Lester 2021, 2). As Johnson and Lester (2021) note, "It is important to recognize that while mental health concerns in academia may be experienced as highly individualized, they are tied to larger structural factors. Changes in higher education structures and governance over the past few decades directly impact faculty and student wellbeing" (2). Neoliberalism, hustle culture, the adjunctification of the workforce, and so on all contribute to a culture of anxiety around higher education.

How do people like me—ambitious, anxious people—survive, let alone thrive, in a culture that pushes all the wrong buttons and feeds our mental disorder? I am still figuring it out. After that stairwell moment and the breakdown that followed, I had to consciously make some decisions about how I wanted to live my life. I chose to step off the tenure track, even though I was eligible for full professor, and change institutions and roles. I am still at an academic institution, working directly with faculty instead of students, and my stress levels are exponentially less than they were before. But I also work with faculty all over the country who are dealing with burnout and anxiety, so I may have changed my situation but not the system that caused it. That work remains to be done by us all.

STIGMA

Stigma: a mark of disgrace associated with a particular circumstance, quality, or person

[TEN]

No One Brought a Casserole

MELISSA NICOLAS

I have bipolar disorder and borderline personality tendencies
I have been a patient in mental hospitals
I am a tenured full professor at an R1 university
I have twice been an associate dean

All of these statements are true
However irreconcilable they seem

When you have struggled with mental health since your childhood, where do you begin the story?

A Day in the Life

As the light from the tall windows streams across her face, I can just make out some sparse patches in her otherwise tightly curled thick hair. She reaches up to scratch her nose, and I see scars up and down her arms. I know that she has been cutting herself, but I cannot ask her that directly, so instead I ask, as innocently as I can, "What happened to your arm?" She knows I know they are from cutting. She also tells me that she has been pulling her hair out, which explains those sparse patches. She has yet to go to the counseling center, and her mom, many hundreds of miles away, is very worried about her. But even her mom does not know about the cutting and the hair pulling. This student is in my office to talk about her failing grades, which seem so beside the point to me right now as I listen to her tell a disjointed story about her mind unraveling.

I am not a counselor; I am an English professor who finds herself as an associate dean in charge of academic support services for a small liberal arts college. It takes over 2 hours, but I finally convince this student to walk with me over to the counseling center. I sit with her there for another 45 minutes until someone infinitely more qualified than me takes over. I have spent close to 3 hours with this one student.

I leave work a little early this day, too spent to even open email. I leave my five-year-old at day care so I can be alone. I collapse on the sofa and stare at the wall, unmoving for over an hour. I get up to go to the refrigerator and cannot bring myself to open it, so I slide down to the floor and prop myself up against it, staring at nothing until my husband gets home with my son. When he sees me, I can tell my husband's face is registering fear, but I do not quite understand why. I have just been sitting on the floor. Is it dark outside now? I thought it was still afternoon.

My husband coaxes me back over to the sofa and switches on the TV. I stare at the moving pictures and listen to the discordant sounds coming from the box as he feeds my son dinner. I am not hungry. At some point—I have no idea how much time is passing—he tells me he is worried about me because I am so checked out. During the past few months, I have either been in a rage or sobbing all the time, but tonight I am just quiet and distant. My face is blank, and my eyes are vacant. He asks me if there is someone I can call.

Who would I call? What would I say? There is nothing on my mind. I am not feeling anything. I just want to sit and stare. We have only recently moved to a new town, so I do not have a therapist or a psychiatrist or even a new primary care doctor. I have no friends in this new place, and my family does not live close by.

I do not want to move, to speak, to expend any energy, but I can tell that something must be wrong because of the way my husband is speaking to me—as if I am a child. And everything is moving in slow motion. Somewhere in the recesses of my mind, I recall that we have some sort of employee assistance program. I spend way more energy than I have finding the number and calling. Because it is after 5:00 p.m., no one there can help me except to give me a list of names and numbers to call the next day. My crisis, apparently, needs to happen within regular business hours. At the end of the call is a suggestion that I call my local hospital. My husband insists I call even though I think it is a waste of time. I am not sick. Why do I need a hospital?

I get connected with someone—a nurse? a social worker? a therapist?—and start explaining how I just do not want to move and just want to stare at things. I am not sad or angry, just numb and exhausted. She suggests I go to the emergency room (ER). I still do not understand why, but she is the nicest person I have talked to in a long time, so I go.

When I get to the ER, a grumpy triage nurse asks me why I am there, and I tell him that the woman I talked to on the phone told me to come. That answer is not good enough for him, and he asks me again why I am there. I tell him the same thing, that the woman I spoke to on the phone thought it would be a good idea to go to the ER and talk to someone. He is still not satisfied with the answer, even though I give him the name of the person who told me to come. He wants me to say what is wrong with me. I tell him that I was just staring at things. Apparently, the ER does not treat staring. He asks me for a third time why I am there and something snaps. I am enveloped with rage and start shouting at him. A security guard comes closer. I lower my voice and say something about having a nervous breakdown, so he types up a hospital ID bracelet, puts it on my wrist, and gruffly tells me to sit and wait. I am no longer just staring at things. Now I am jumpy, agitated. I want to pace, but the security guard is creeping me out.

It will be two weeks before I go home.

* * *

In clinical terms, according to the *Diagnostic and Statistical Manual V*, my diagnoses have been severe anxiety, clinical depression (mild, moderate, severe), bipolar II, and borderline personality tendencies. My therapist is always quick to remind me that "borderline tendencies" are not the same as having "real" borderline personality disorder, so I guess I should say that too, right? Because that makes some kind of difference to someone—the insurance company, probably.

I am a card-carrying member of the Prozac Nation, having been on some form of psychotropic meds since my early 20s—various and sundry antidepressants, antianxiety meds, and mood stabilizers.

Over the course of my adult life, I have spent about 2 weeks in a mental hospital. The first stay was about 10 days and the second stay about 3 days. They happened about 10 years apart.

Along the way I have been tenured four times due to changing institutions multiple times and being promoted to full professor. Until quite recently, most people, both colleagues and friends, did not know the extent of my mental health history. Sometimes I would vaguely refer to depression or join in reciting the agony woes of being overstressed and overworked, which everyone on the tenure track feels. Still, it was rare that I would let people know, especially people who had any say over my career, just *how* depressed I was.

But Were You Really Sick?

Six months after my first hospital stay and one month after the completion of an intensive outpatient program, I return to work. I am worried that people will know I have been in a mental hospital and will be judging my fitness to be back in the office, but I am not quite prepared for the stories I do encounter. The predominant narrative seems to be that I had a brain tumor and died; I guess they think they are seeing a ghost. But this makes sense on a very basic level. Right before I went out on disability, I was having horrible migraine attacks. People knew about those attacks because there was no shame in leaving work for those. I would tell the dean and my office assistant and colleagues that I was leaving early because my head hurt. Headaches are acceptable. Indeed, given my position, no one seemed especially surprised that I was having migraines. My job was a stressful one to be sure.

The other common narrative is that I had some kind of cancer and no one knew whether I would be returning to work. I guess that makes some sense as well, since I left rather suddenly and no one saw me much after that. And I suppose cancer is more palatable than the truth because, while dying from cancer would have made for a tragic story, cancer is just bad luck (she was so young!). A broken mind hits too close to home.

Even though these are the stories acknowledged publicly, I am not back too long before I hear the whispers. Of course there are whispers. I am at a small college where everyone knows everyone, and I my position was high profile.

At first I think I am paranoid (I mean, I am mentally unbalanced, right?). How could people know I am struggling with mental health if no one truly knows where I have been? But the pieces start falling into place quickly: If people thought I had died, why had no one reached out to my husband? We lived in faculty housing on campus. No one so much as brought him a casserole or homemade muffins. And my son, who attends the campus day care, has been showing up for school. At least his class made me some Get Well cards. I received nothing from my colleagues—no flowers, no cards, no chocolates.

There were no meal trains like when my colleague had cancer, no home visits, no offers to help with my son. People knew. I was contaminated. I had the illness whose name we dare not speak. Maybe people were afraid it was contagious. One day I was at work doing my very difficult job, and the next day I was gone with no clear explanations.

As time passes and I work to make sense of what happened, I am struck by the silence surrounding it.

There was my silence, of course. I chose not to divulge what was happening to me. And for quite a long time, I believed my decision to not be forthcoming about what I was going through was the reason for so much secrecy surrounding my absence. But as time has passed, I have begun to see things a little differently.

Why, for example, did I feel I needed to keep silent? What were the unspoken but very audible messages I received from the institution that frightened me into secrecy? Why did I feel as though my career would be over (even though I was tenured, a privileged position to begin with) if people knew I had a mental illness, not a physical one? Why did no one reach out?

Legally, when you go out on disability leave, your job, or its equivalent, must be waiting for you when you get back. My university played a little fast and loose with this. My dean said, "You are a tenured member of the faculty, so you always have a home here." But my position as associate dean was a little more tenuous. Obviously, while I was out, someone had to step in as interim to take my place—the students did not stop needing help just because I was out. The person who took over as interim had never particularly liked the way I had done the job to begin with, so she was quite happy, I think, to get in there and shake some things up.

Given the trauma I had been through, I did not especially want to return to my position in the same capacity I had been in when I left, so I asked for some accommodations to lighten the workload. I was told, however, that that was impossible. But because I did not specifically ask not to return to my dean's role, the university could not refuse to allow me to come back to the dean's office. So they kept the interim position going and then redefined the scope of the job to include duties I had never done. I was then told I could reapply for my job. All this is technically legal. But it was crummy. And I found out after the fact that during the discussions of my candidacy for my old position, my leave of absence came up as a reason I should not be considered. This discussion, of course, is illegal. But I was too tired, too burned out, still too fragile to really fight them on this. At this point I decided it was time to leave the institution.

In many ways I feel as though I left with my tail between my legs, going from associate dean to pariah to persona non grata. When people would see us in the parking lot in faculty housing, they would put their heads down and hurry into their houses or otherwise ignore us. When I went into my department office building to pick up some things from my office, one of my colleagues saw me and literally turned away from the door so she did not have to acknowledge me. I was gaslighted before it was a thing.

When I began my new job at a new institution, I was scared to death of anyone finding out what had happened to me at my last job. And I was on high alert for any internal signals or hints that I was headed down the road to hospitalization again.

Hello, Skeleton

The scars of this experience have stayed with me, and while we certainly do talk about mental health in the academy more today than we did 10 years ago, it is still not okay to actually have mental health issues that go beyond taking some antidepressants. When I needed to be hospitalized recently, the same kind of shame and silence surrounded that event. The department was told that I was out sick—which is technically true—but no one was told what was happening. This time I was only out of work for about 8 days—3 days in a horrible hospital (which is a story for a different time) and about 5 days trying to put my life back together at home.

I made the decision this time, though, that I was not going to keep quiet about where I was or what had happened because there was nothing to be ashamed of. So I told my department chair the whole saga. And then I told some of my work friends. And, finally, I came out to my students. I admitted to them that I had experienced a mental health crisis and gotten help and was working on healing.

I was petrified to do this because I had no idea of the impact this disclosure would have on my relationships with my students or colleagues. As it turns out, I did not need to worry so much. My students were overwhelmingly supportive, caring, and concerned. Some asked if there was anything they could do for me. Others, some in the moment, some many months later, admitted that it felt kind of good that someone whom they saw as successful (me, their tenured professor with a doctorate) has struggles similar to theirs.

But I still wonder: Why do we continue to talk in hushed tones and whispers about mental health in the academy? Why does it feel like a "coming out" to admit that we have issues? Why do I still caution my own graduate students about divulging their mental health struggles too publicly before they land a permanent job? Maybe it is generational, and things are slowly changing. My students are definitely more open about their mental health issues than those in my generation. But being in the academy as a professional, being lauded and paid for what your mind can do, is a fraught position when your mind is suspect.

If *your* mind is suspect, then *anyone*'s mind could be suspect. And that is a truth we would still rather not acknowledge in the academy.

ELEVEN

Alone at the Table

Neurodivergence and Fractured Networks

RONNIE K. STEPHENS

THE PRESSURE TO DEVELOP professional networks is one of the most pervasive hallmarks in higher education, a pressure embedded in faculty contracts and perpetually reinforced by the culture of academia. Professional advancement depends not just on our ability to present at conferences and publish in peer-reviewed spaces but also on our ability to position ourselves alongside other scholars in our respective fields. Additionally, many institutions have faculty recognition practices predicated on nomination and support from colleagues within the department, emphasizing the need to develop networks both outside our home campuses and within our departments. Failure to effectively network can stand in the way of promotions, appointments, and applications for tenure.

Though I have been tangentially aware that my struggles to navigate social spaces affect my ability to form professional networks, the consequences were never more clear than when I applied for advancement in rank during my fourth year with my current institution. Despite exceptional evaluations from my dean and a strong record of praise from my department chair, my application was denied because I was "not visible enough" at the institution. I had met every professional and academic requirement for advancement, yet I was passed over because I rarely attended events on campus or optional faculty gatherings. My avoidance of such events is a direct result of living with schizoid personality disorder (SPD), a condition that makes it nearly impossible for me to correctly process social cues and causes such extreme social anxiety that my diagnostician recommended I self-isolate for six to eight hours after *any* social engagement. While I was dejected by the decision to deny my application, I was hardly surprised; I have struggled to assimilate to academic spaces for as long as I can remember.

Early Experience

My troubled relationship with academia began almost immediately. Near the close of my kindergarten year, my teacher and principal both advised that I should forgo entering first grade and instead enter what was then termed "developmental first grade." The purpose of this interlude was purportedly to assist students who were not emotionally prepared for first grade and to give them more time to, in their words, "mature." Two things happened as a direct result of my year in developmental first grade: First, the mandated group therapy sessions triggered a lifelong discomfort with therapeutic settings, and second, my predilection for academic study put me further ahead of my peers. There was, unfortunately, no measurable improvement in my ability to socialize with people my age. The end result was that I continued to feel alienated in first grade, though that alienation grew to include not just my peer group but also my teacher, who was so determined to get me to ask questions during class that she began assigning me work increasingly beyond the first-grade curriculum. I did not ask her a single question that year, even as I worked through fifth-grade math and language arts textbooks. She viewed this refusal as an act of defiance, an attitude that colored my reputation among teachers all the way to graduation. Despite a near obsession with learning and continually high marks in class, I hated school.

Grad School Realizations

During my first year of graduate school, I was forced to confront my underlying disdain for educators because a teaching assistantship had become available that would offset tuition costs. Numerous peers and adults throughout my undergraduate career had encouraged me to consider teaching given my talent and willingness to help friends prepare for exams, guide others through mutual assignments, and explain challenging concepts. Though I have always loved learning and enjoyed talking about coursework with peers, my experiences with teachers throughout adolescence drove me to dismiss their advice on every front. After all, my teachers had been chastising me for working alone and failing to assimilate to group work since first grade, some going so far as to tell me that I would never amount to anything and would never succeed in life if I could not learn to work with others. Still, a teaching assistantship would provide financial benefits that I desperately needed, so I accepted and began my first course on pedagogy the following semester.

The course encouraged frequent group work and collective study sessions, and every teaching assistant was paired with a tenured faculty member who would act as a mentor for our first semesters teaching both Composition I and Composition II. I had come to accept my near-constant sense of isolation, which, most of the time, was actually a source of comfort. Working in close proximity to others, as a student or a teacher, caused me extreme anxiety and frustration. Several of my peers in the pedagogy course accepted my idiosyncrasies and treated me with kindness. They frequently invited me to gatherings and even suggested I host our end-of-semester study session because I was more comfortable in my own space.

Looking back, one thing that stands out is how emotionally connected I felt to numerous colleagues even though I knew almost nothing about them and never engaged any of them in conversation beyond our shared study. When I left the program, I lost contact with all of them, something that had already become a theme in my personal and professional relationships. Through the clarity of my diagnosis, I now understand that I often misconstrue comfort with an individual and kindness in daily interactions as markers of friendship, yet I struggle with the concept of maintaining relationships with individuals. I was not actually close to my colleagues but felt drawn to them out of familiarity. Though we might have been friends after the program, I failed to maintain individual relationships in the absence of forced or structured interactions. The most isolating aspect of this dynamic is that I felt a deep admiration and kinship with several of my colleagues, yet I could not follow through on expected social conventions and gave the impression that I was not invested in them outside the structure of the program.

Teaching for America

Various life circumstances caused me to pivot away from education in 2008, and I briefly entered a career researching mineral rights for an oil and gas conglomerate. The job was perfect because I worked entirely alone and spent my entire work day doing research. I felt more invigorated and balanced than I ever had. While lucrative, the foray was short-lived as the recession and housing market crash forced my employer to reduce labor. Jobs were limited for the remainder of 2008, and I soon found myself in an alternative certification program for secondary education. After my experiences as a teaching assistant, the idea of being a teacher full-time felt more rewarding and exciting, but I quickly ran into a problem: every school district I encountered required at least one year of experience. After a year of applications and interviews, I found an inroad in Teach for America (TFA).

I knew nothing about the organization other than the fact that they brought on teachers with no experience and often accepted people who came to education through nontraditional paths. In hindsight I could not have been a worse fit for the organization, which is composed almost entirely of ambitious individuals who see TFA as an opportunity to grow networks for future careers outside the classroom. I was the exact opposite; I had no desire to network and no ambition outside being an effective educator. I encountered problems with my peers, mentors, and administration before I had even completed their summer training institute. Many of those drawn to the organization were extroverted and comfortable with networking events; my tendency to avoid optional gatherings and remain relatively quiet in group settings again gave the impression that I was not invested in others or interested in building relationships. Peers quickly decided not to invite me to after-hours events, and mentors began to pull me aside to discuss my perceived lack of commitment to the organization. By the end of my first year with TFA, I was alienated to the point that only two members of the organization spoke to me, and one of them was my assigned mentor.

For me, the most frustrating part of my alienation within TFA was that I exceeded their goals and expectations at every turn. The organization is remarkably fixated on standardized testing, data-driven pedagogy, and measurable results. I embraced their methods with vigor and immersed myself in improving the literacy of my students, and according to the various assessments TFA required me to implement, my students were growing well beyond expectations. My administrators consistently praised my ability to connect with students and heighten their understanding, often openly planning schedules and rosters so that struggling students were in my sections. I was thriving in the classroom and had strong relationships with my students, yet again I was entirely alienated from my colleagues both on campus and in the TFA.

This alienation was grounded not in my teaching effectiveness but in my inability to build strong networks. I had not distinguished myself among peers for one simple reason: I failed to build interpersonal relationships. From their perspective I was unwilling to invest in them the way that I invested in students. What I could not understand or communicate at the time is that people with SPD generally thrive in relationships with large age gaps because there is a clear power dynamic that helps dictate expected social interactions.

Diagnosis

Four years into my teaching career, I moved to a new state where teacher salaries were considerably higher and raising a family more tenable. I hoped for a fresh start and better relationships with my colleagues, but the trend of success in the classroom and alienation among peers continued. After eight years of teaching high school, my wife and I agreed that public education was not the right fit and that my inability to develop functional relationships with others in the profession would likely be a constant source of discord. So after completing a master of fine arts degree, I put all my energy into teaching at the college level. Within a year, I held a full-time post with a community college; my administration was excited to bring me on as a dual-credit instructor given my experience in secondary education and my ability to connect with high school students.

Ironically, one of the most immediate changes with my new position was my access to an insurance provider who covered screenings for autism and other mental health diagnoses. At the time we had been trying to locate a diagnostician to work with one of our children, who showed various and increasing signs of autism. After learning that my new insurance provider would cover the screening, we proceeded, and our child was, in fact, diagnosed with autism spectrum disorder (ASD). My wife, after reading our child's diagnostic report, suggested that I pursue a screening for myself because, she said, many of the descriptors in the report sounded like me. I agreed and, though I was already in my mid-30s, set up a screening for myself.

My diagnostician administered a battery of tests and surveys over the course of five hours, which, oddly, felt very stimulating for me. The following week she called me in to discuss her findings: of the markers for ASD, she found that I exhibited all of them except one, cognitive flexibility. She explained that my having cognitive flexibility was a disqualifying factor for an ASD diagnosis, so I was not on the spectrum. Based on the remaining indicators, however, she offered the diagnosis of schizoid personality disorder, depression, and generalized anxiety disorder (GAD). Neither depression nor GAD surprised me given my years of suicidal ideation and extreme aversion to social interactions. What was most enlightening, though, is that she described my mental health diagnoses as directly linked to SPD. Essentially, having SPD correlated with my inability to read social cues, form relationships with members of my peer group, and process emotion in a healthy manner. In fact, my diagnostician recommended no fewer than six to eight hours of complete isolation following any social interaction. Failing to do so, she warned, could lead to intensified feelings of depression and anxiety. Total isolation was and is impossible, of course; together, my wife and I have six children and live in a multigenerational home. I am, quite frankly, never alone.

One of the other recommendations included in my diagnostic report was to avoid social interactions whenever possible, which is a difficult recommendation to adhere to in light of my chosen profession. Still, understanding more about how daily interactions can and do trigger anxiety offered an opportunity to better prepare myself for the many ways in which my career requires me to work closely with others. As I learned more about navigating life with SPD, I also gained insight into why I was routinely able to connect with my students but not my peers. As it happens, the social dynamics involved in relationships with people much younger or much older than myself help to offset many of the anxieties that manifest in relationships with peers. I am, it seems, uniquely skilled at interacting with students but woefully challenged with regard to networking and developing professional relationships.

The Need for Networks

Unfortunately for me, networking is integral to career advancement in higher education. Catherine Armstrong (Shaw 2013), a senior lecturer in American history at Manchester Metropolitan University, explained in an interview with Claire Shaw of *The Guardian* that "networking on both a formal and informal level . . . is vital for any academic who wants to develop his or her career." Christian Teeter (2020) likewise argues that professional networks enhance the value of higher education degrees and improve socioeconomic status in his essay "Professional Networks within U.S. Higher Education: Avenues to Foster Career and Institutional Success." Jarrod Sadulski (2021), in his essay "Higher Education Networking during the COVID-19 Pandemic," further reinforces the importance of networking in academia and how limited access to physical conferences during the pandemic may have had a negative impact on career academics.

The need for strong professional networks in higher education is not a secret, but the impact of my mental health and SPD on my academic career, financial livelihood, and professional network was far less obvious until very recently. Like most higher education institutions, my college has a specific process in place for promotions in rank and tenure. Tenure is treated as the more rigorous of the processes, while promotions in rank generally correlate with academic achievement. When I was hired, the college deemed me six credits shy of the assistant professor rank. As part of my personal and professional commitment to the field, I decided to pursue a PhD in English from a local university, a plan approved by each tier of administration before I began. From 2020 to 2022, I completed all necessary coursework and comprehensive exams, advancing to the "all but dissertation" stage with a 4.0 in the program. Having completed the requisite three-year probationary period at my college and earned the necessary hours, I compiled the mandatory materials to apply for promotion in rank to assistant professor.

Despite meeting and exceeding every marker for promotion, the vice president elected not to advance my application to the board. Her reasoning: I had not distinguished myself as an asset to the college on the basis that I did not have a strong presence at social functions or broad professional relationships with my colleagues. The most frustrating part of this, for me, is that the vice president explicitly dismissed my professional achievements as selfish pursuits that detracted from my service to the college. Over my first three years with the college, I had presented at almost a dozen conferences, published numerous academic articles, placed chapters in four academic collections, and established myself as a staff reviewer of poetry for a national publication. Almost all this work was done in pursuit of the one thing higher education professionals must curate: networks.

Perhaps understandably, my first reaction to being denied a promotion in rank was frustration. I felt slighted and overlooked, triggering memories of a fraught relationship to academia from kindergarten forward. For the first time, though, I had access to my diagnosis; that information proved vital as I tried to process the news and move forward in my current position. I thought back to each conference I had attended, each professional development week with my college, and my relationship with peers in my PhD program. Across all of these spaces, I was ostensibly taking steps to build a robust network. Though I put myself in the right spaces and excelled at the individual level, what I came to realize is how drastically my SPD was affecting my ability to build relationships.

At conference after conference, the only time I spoke was to present a paper and field questions during my scheduled panel. I attended panels excitedly, brimming with questions about the research I heard and jotting notes in my spiral, only to quietly slip out from the back row without a word. During professional development sessions and faculty luncheons at my college, I routinely brought a book and sat deliberately away from my peers as much as possible. In my PhD courses, I participated eagerly, yet I spoke almost exclusively to my professors. At every turn I dismissed invitations to social events, often using my family as a scapegoat when in reality I felt constantly drained by the myriad expectations of social interaction just to get through my professional and academic commitments. Interacting outside what was absolutely necessary seemed impossible, even as I harbored continued feelings of alienation that pushed me deeper into depression. I wanted (and want) desperately to engage with fellow literature enthusiasts and passionate educators, but doing so (or planning to do so) regularly induces panic attacks. And for the first time in my higher education career, I understand that I may always be alone at the table, consistently exceeding expectations in the classroom and disappearing into the shadows of my colleagues on campus.

Important Reads

This realization is damning and defeatist, I know, but it also reinvigorated me to improve as an educator. It seems inevitable that continued improvement in the classroom will not necessarily correlate with professional advancement, but the stuff of teaching has always given me life in a way that professional advancement simply does not. To combat the overwhelming sense of despair associated with the relative stagnation of my career, I shifted my focus to my students and to deeper dives into contemporary pedagogy. Surprisingly, I have encountered only a handful of pedagogical texts that directly address mental health in higher education and what professors can do to navigate neurodivergence in their respective careers. While the research may be minimal at present, two books in particular have proven indispensable in my practice.

The first is Jessamyn Neuhaus's (2019) *Geeky Pedagogy*, a remarkable book that offers concrete praxis to circumvent the challenges of being a neurodivergent educator. Among them, Neuhaus encourages neurodivergent educators to deliberately block off time during class to engage students in dialogue outside the content of the course. Since many neurodivergent educators struggle with social cues and building relationships, planning for social interaction both ensures that we make time to connect with our students as individuals and alleviates some of the anxiety around unstructured dialogue. She further stresses that teaching and learning are a social interaction, not a transaction. As I read *Geeky Pedagogy*, I realized that a fundamental failure in all my attempts to network was that I viewed the process as entirely transactional. I sought to exchange ideas and professional growth with peers, rather than to build relationships with them as human beings. This is a by-product of SPD, but knowing the terminology and understanding behind the process is a vital step in learning how to work against my natural instinct to self-isolate.

Another book essential to bridging my mental health with my career is Christopher Schaberg's (2022) *Pedagogy of the Depressed*, in which Schaberg centers the mental health of both educators and students. Like Neuhaus, and virtually every contemporary academic writing about pedagogy, he emphasizes the importance of restoring humanity in the classroom. Doing so, he argues, will not only reduce anxiety in our students but also help offset depression in educators because we are fixated less on measurable outputs and more on human connection. It is sometimes jarringly simple to fail at teaching content, but it is almost impossible to fail our students if we prioritize connecting with them on a human level.

I would love to end this chapter with a message of hope or some example of how my diagnosis has fundamentally improved my professional networks. The truth is, it has not, at least not yet. Most days I still struggle with intense depression and loneliness. I know with absolute certainty that when I return to campus for the coming semester, I will select back rows and corner seats far from my peers. In a few months, I will present at yet another conference and more than likely speak only for the duration of my panel. One thing has changed, though: I have learned to give myself the same grace that I offer my students. I am learning to see myself, like my students, as someone with unique and persistent needs that make mundane social situations feel overwhelming. As Walt Whitman once wrote, "I celebrate myself, and sing myself." And these days, I have a few more terms for the chorus, a little more clarity about my song, and a tad more confidence in the way that I sing.

TWELVE

Don't Ask Me How I'm Doing

LEE SKALLERUP BESSETTE

TODAY WAS SUPPOSED to be a day when I went into the office, but instead I have to pick up the youngest from school and stay home with them. Again. I am grateful for my job and that my colleagues are so understanding of my need to work remotely a lot more than my hybrid job designation would otherwise indicate. But I wonder when that grace will wear out. I long for the freedom to go back to the office more regularly, but I also dread the small talk that comes from being there. People ask how I am doing, and it is either a bald-faced lie or I run away before dissolving into tears.

In the past year, my youngest child (14) has been hospitalized twice, stayed in a residential mental health care facility across the country from us, and received an autism diagnosis. My oldest (16) has been diagnosed with a number of chronic illnesses and had to give up their passion because they were physically no longer able to participate. They suffer from anxiety and attention deficit hyperactivity disorder (ADHD), plus dealing with the stress of what their sibling is going through. They are close in age (21 months apart) and close in relationship. The oldest swears that they love the youngest the best out of all the family.

I wear my stress on my body as extra weight. Now I worry that when I get into the office people will notice, and my internalized fat phobia rears its ugly head—another thing to add to the list of reasons I am bad. I am a bad person for letting myself go, so to speak. I am a bad parent for letting the autism go unnoticed for so long. I am a bad parent for letting my oldest stay home from school so often. I am a bad parent for having sent the youngest away. I am a bad employee for having to work from home so much. I am a bad person for letting self-care fall to the wayside. I am a bad feminist for taking on so much of this burden because my husband's job is more demanding, pays more, and is where the insurance is coming from.

I started writing about my own struggles with mental health issues over a decade ago. I wrote about my depression for the *University of Venus* blog at *Inside Higher Ed* (Bessette 2012), with subsequent follow-ups on my own personal blog and then the *College Ready Writing* blog at *Inside Higher Ed*. I did a series called "Bad Female Academic" (Bessette 2011), which I described as follows:

> Every week, I will look at all the ways I am a Bad Female Academic. Some weeks, it will be about why I am a bad academic more generally, sometimes about how I am a bad female. Other weeks, it will be why I am a bad combination of the two. I specifically want to deal with the ways in which our communities (large and small) try to limit who I am and how I am allowed to view and understand myself. The pressures academia places on me are well-known, as are larger societal messages about who I am supposed to be as a woman, mother, and wife. When these two worlds collide . . .

Since then I have been diagnosed with ADHD, which explains a lot of what I was writing about (and against) over the past decade. I used to hold up my status as a Bad Female Academic as something to be proud of, of being different in a good way, of going against the grain of what academia would have me be.

I have subsequently started a podcast with a colleague on being a neurodivergent Generation X woman in academia, and my work within the institution has been heavily informed by my own lived experience. I work in a teaching and learning center where I take the issues of accessibility and inclusivity very seriously. I have also overhauled my own personal pedagogy. With everything I have learned, I foolishly thought that I could at least mitigate, if not avoid, the struggles I have been through by parenting differently from how both my husband and I were parented.

It is hard for me to even picture how things could be worse than they have been. This was the best we could do?

I am extraordinarily privileged, and not just because I have a job that is flexible enough that I can work from home. We are white and middle class, so my children, rather than being labeled troublemakers, were dealt with carefully and with understanding for the most part in school. We have excellent insurance. We could afford to fly across the country at a moment's notice because our youngest was no longer safe at home. Our school district has really great alternative schooling options for both our oldest and youngest. The youngest's team at their middle school has been wonderful and compassionate and patient and supportive.

And yet I still feel like I am drowning.

Because we have moved around so much for our (academic) jobs (did we move too much?) and the pandemic (do not even get me started on what impact that had), we do not have a robust support network (is it because we are not modeling healthy social relationships or cutting them off from "the village" model of parenting?). It gets easier and easier to cut off the potential support I do have as we move further along because the more complicated this all gets, the more I must explain to fill anyone in on just what we need (I do not even know anymore) and why we need it (please do not judge me or my kids).

What I need is to not have a major executive functioning disorder that makes it hard to do all the little things that must be done, like paying the medical bills; keeping track of what has been billed, been paid, or is outstanding; who needs a new doctor; what meds need refilling; what forms need to be filled out; where and when these forms should be submitted, on top of the "normal" things a parent (okay, mother) needs to keep track of. The oldest unloaded on me recently, torn between understanding that I have a lot on my plate and needing my attention to help them find a new activity and get in to see more doctors.

I hesitate to dig deeply into the research literature on the mental health of parents of kids with autism (spoiler: not great!) or the mental health of the siblings of said child with autism (spoiler: also not great!). It all seems futile at times. Speaking to an expert who helps match kids with mental health issues with an appropriate treatment facility (a.k.a. therapeutic boarding school), I despair that what we have already done is probably not enough. There is also no way we can afford the level of care that is probably needed (why did I choose academia?).

And yet. I show up to work almost every day, although I have been better about taking days off as mental health breaks. My work gets done. I teach my class, do my consultations, develop and deliver my workshops, attend my meetings, do my part, and do it well. I cannot remember names all that well right now, and if it is not on my calendar, I will most certainly forget it, but mostly, I do a good job at appearing to be normal. My husband reached out to a colleague whose own child struggled with mental health issues, and the colleague marveled at how well we are dealing with our situation and how they never could have, only having to deal with [insert another different but equally difficult and challenging situation that we cannot imagine having to deal with].

When you are in it, all you can do is keep going.

I feel like a fraud. I know that one kind person, one understanding instructor, can make all the difference in the life of a student, and so I keep offering workshops and doing consultations about inclusivity, compassion, trauma-informed pedagogy, and accessibility. But I also know that none of that will ultimately really help my kids if and when they get to college; that what they need is something more than the university can provide for them and that society is willing to provide for them, for us, for me.

We keep hearing about the staff shortages in higher education, and I have to believe that the increase in the number of children struggling with mental health issues is part of the reason, disproportionately affecting women who drop out of the workforce to care for their kids. I cherish the flexibility I do have and the understanding my team has shown me because if not for that, I am not sure I would have been able to stay in the workforce.

But also, I cannot afford to leave, either.

Therapists are too few, everything is too expensive, everything takes too much time, mental illness and chronic conditions do not follow a schedule or set timeline. . . . Everyone, including my employer, is doing everything they can, and it still is not enough.

My therapist recommended an app, called Mindfulness Bell, that goes off at a random point every waking hour. When it does, I am to take three deep breaths and say, on the inhale, "I am ok" and, on the exhale, "I can do this." It works remarkably well, and she tells me that soldiers with post-traumatic stress disorder also find it quite effective. All my body knows now are trauma responses.

I am learning that my worth is not wrapped up in how productive I am nor how "well" I parent. Years ago, when my youngest was first (mis)diagnosed as having ADHD, we had a conversation about the difference between privacy (something you do not want widely known) and secrets (something you feel ashamed to share). It was a heavy conversation with an eight-year-old dealing with something they thought they should be ashamed of or embarrassed about. I am trying to remind myself of that truth in these moments and as I write this piece. I want to protect my kids' privacy and do not want to feel embarrassed or ashamed for sharing.

I am constantly and annoyingly asking my kids if they are okay and how they are doing. I have become fine-tuned to their responses. I want them to be honest with me, even if they are trying to protect my feelings. I try to be as honest as I can with them about how I am feeling, how things are going with me, without unfairly burdening them. I stopped going to therapy because I would spend the entire session telling my therapist just how badly the past week had gone, and when she asked me what I needed, I was at a loss. I need things to get easier.

At my annual evaluation at work, I took a step back and looked at all I had accomplished professionally this past year even with all of this other stuff going on. I marked myself as having been "outstanding" in all categories only because "heroic" was not an option. I could not celebrate my accomplishments because it did not seem appropriate, but downplaying everything also seemed dishonest. I was outstanding. I was also terrible.

Working on my evaluation, I realized my priorities have dramatically shifted. *Of course* my priorities have shifted. So many of us working in higher education have shifted our priorities when faced with our own or a loved one's mental or physical health struggles. Many, as I alluded to earlier, have chosen to leave. I have decided to forcefully assert a work-life balance, which can run afoul of the cult of productivity that runs through not just higher education but our society writ large. I have started saying no. I have started asking for what I need, rather than contorting myself to work in settings optimized for neurotypicals. I have stopped apologizing for resting.

I can still do excellent work without looking like I am working hard, if that makes sense. I did not have the energy to look like I was working hard at work because I was too busy trying to make it look like everything was okay. I can only wear one mask at a time, so the mask of "everything is okay" replaced the "look at how hard I am working" mask. But for many of us, even just one mask is too much these days, and so we let them fall. I am not sure anyone is ready, however, for a chorus of us revealing who we really are and demanding what we need to feel like we belong.

I need people to stop asking me how I am doing. I am doing fine. I am doing awful. I am doing more than I ever thought I would be able to and then some. Surprisingly good but also dreadful.

THIRTEEN

My Autistic Transformation

A Journey Toward Acceptance and Advocacy

DIXIE L. BURNS

IN THE BEGINNING of the fall 2023 semester, I was completely open for the first time to all my students and colleagues about my neurodivergent status. Standing in front of my classroom, nerves and overwhelm struggled against my desire to be an advocate for change. Over this past year, I have been sharing with some colleagues and students, and the relief from other neurodivergent individuals as they realize they are not alone has led me to realize I can do more. This is the next step on my journey in combating stigmas against neurodivergent conditions and mental health issues. A part of me wants to continue hiding, yet I feel strongly that this is something I must do to give meaning to my past struggles and help create a more inclusive future for all of us.

I am autistic. I was officially diagnosed at nearly 50. I also have co-occurring conditions of generalized anxiety disorder (GAD), obsessive-compulsive disorder (OCD), sensory processing disorder (SPD), and prosopagnosia (face blindness). I have difficulty in social situations relating to and understanding others. I often fail to comprehend others' emotions or read their nonverbal cues, then I am confused when people react. I often feel misunderstood and isolated. I have a strong attachment to routines and patterns and become agitated when things do not go according to plan. I am often uncomfortable with eye contact and struggle with recognizing faces. Sometimes I am bothered by casual physical touch or being too close to people. I am very sensitive to loud noises and bright lights. All of this creates constant anxiety for me as I try to blend in.

I have always known I was different, but for much of my life I did not know why. I struggled to fit in and understand the world around me, yet I always remained on the outside. I have spent so much time trying to be normal and continually feeling like there is something wrong with me. I feel like a square peg trying to fit into a world of round holes.

Struggling to Appear Normal

From childhood on I was clearly different. I struggled to appear "normal." Unfortunately, in the 1970s and 1980s autism was not widely diagnosed and recognized, especially if you were smart and quiet and female. Nobody could identify what was wrong with me, yet everyone seemed to know I was not normal. It seemed I was failing to pay attention: I would "zone out" and was in my own world. My hearing was tested, and nothing was wrong there. I did not speak right—my voice was too monotone, so I underwent speech therapy. I walked funny and was klutzy. I did not look people in the eye. I fidgeted too much and would not sit still. On and on the list went.

Growing up on a small Wisconsin dairy farm, I spent my early childhood alone in the outdoors. My first encounters with my peers were in elementary school. Entering kindergarten was a shock. My life changed abruptly as I was suddenly thrust into a group of strangers and forced into a different environment and routine. I did not fit; I was not normal or typical. I quickly became isolated from my peers, and unfortunately this began years of my being a victim of bullying. This also began my journey of withdrawal and trying to be invisible. I started to build my mask: suppressing my natural tendencies, my confusion, and my emotions and trying to figure out how I was supposed to act.

I had my first experience with autistic burnout and depression at age 13, although I did not know what it was at the time. I struggled with the transition between elementary and middle school and growing up in general. I felt exhausted, misunderstood, and broken. I physically withdrew from the world, hiding under the covers of my bed, refusing to go to school, and claiming I was ill. I thought about suicide, going as far as to plan where and how. Thankfully, my fear of death was stronger than my fear of the world. I remember visiting medical doctors and overhearing one doctor telling my mother that nothing was physically wrong with me and maybe I needed to see a psychiatrist if things did not improve. This terrified me as I knew a psychiatrist would see how abnormal I really was and lock me up in an institution. While irrational, this fear did motivate me to pretend I was normal and go through the motions of life. I was smart and I was going to use that to fool everyone. I focused on my academics, participated in sports, hid the real "broken" me from the world, and projected the image of a geeky scholar athlete. I decided I was going to be the smartest and use that to get away from small-town America.

By the time I started college at the University of Wisconsin-Madison, I was good at masking and could pass as relatively normal. In situations where my awkwardness came through, I tried to play it up as an odd personality trait. Still, I knew I was not normal. I finally had friends, but I always seemed to be on the outside of my friend groups. Socializing and fitting in was so hard and exhausting, yet everyone else made it seem so easy. I never managed to get along well with my roommates in college. Sharing a dorm my first year and having no space to retreat to was debilitating, yet when I reached out, I was told it was typical adjusting-to-college stuff. I had an easier time when I got my own room in housing, but I still struggled with housemates and fitting in. I once again leaned into my academics, in particular my science and math classes, where there seemed to be a clear logic and order.

Graduate school increased the challenge for me. I was in a new place (Ohio State University), and suddenly, my previous coping skills were not working. I did not understand the networking and social structure; I once again did not know how to fit in. I was constantly in the same building under the same noisy fluorescent lights sharing an office with other busy graduate students. And as a graduate student, I was expected to put in long hours there, so it felt like there was no relief from the constant sensory input. How did others make it so easy? I often felt like I had no idea what I was doing or supposed to be doing. I felt adrift without structure and guidance, yet whenever I sought help and asked questions, the answer always seemed to be "Figure it out for yourself."

I did enjoy being a teaching assistant for the undergrad classes. I was able to talk about my special interest at length. I was good at explaining astronomy to others, but I was also told I spent too much of my time there and needed to manage my time better. I struggled with the narrow focus of research and my inability to see its purpose as I spent hours and days reviewing computer code—something that really did not capture my interest.

As I tried to navigate the politics and interpersonal relationships of graduate school while maintaining my masking, I experienced my second major autistic burnout. Competition for jobs in academia can be intense, and I worried about being able to compete when others made it look so easy. Not understanding why I struggled so much compared to everyone else and feeling misunderstood and avoided by my peers, I left graduate school with my master's degree along with a lot of confusion, extreme exhaustion, and a sense of failure.

I returned to Wisconsin to recover from burnout, put my life back together, and figure out what I wanted to do next. I decided to focus on teaching since I enjoyed talking about all kinds of science, and I had learned in graduate school that I excelled at explaining things. I thought maybe this was a way to make a difference. And I could return to the familiarity of an academic environment. I was hired as an adjunct instructor at Madison Area Technical College, our local community college, in 1998 and became full-time in 2000. Was this finally a place where I could fit in? Could I strengthen my mask and reinvent myself so my new colleagues would think I was normal?

Here I fight imposter syndrome as I try to figure out the role I am supposed to play and how to play it, all the while wondering why I struggle in simple areas when others do not. I am stressed from attempting to hide my deficiencies. As much as I love my job, it drains my energy.

Discovering I Am Autistic yet Still Hiding

Around 2000, during a staff training event, I learned that more and more students with mental disabilities were being mainstreamed into grades K–12. The facilitator wanted us to be aware of some new students with autism who were entering our college and were "different from normal people." As she went on with describing these individuals, I felt more and more like I understood and that I was one of these "different people." They did not seem so odd to me. Perhaps I was autistic.

I began researching autism and self-diagnosed shortly after this. I researched further on ways for autistic people to appear normal. When I taught autistic students with accommodations, I tried to adapt those accommodations to myself so I could function more efficiently. I was determined to keep my autism a secret because it was clear to me from the 2000 training and my research that a stigma was associated with the condition. Years of research about autism and ways to blend in so others did not find out followed.

Health issues finally started catching up with me (again, I suspect autistic burnout). I felt like I was losing control of my life, yet I was so exhausted all the time. I was struggling to maintain my masking, yet I had been doing it so long that I could not be sure who I was without it. I fought to clearly articulate my needs, often weakly expressing them as wants, and of course, they were discounted with statements like "Everyone experiences stress" and "Well, we can't have everything we want all the time." Then came the headaches, nausea, and physical aches and pains as I tried to push through being normal. I felt truly broken and ashamed of my lack of coping skills compared to everyone else, yet a part of me knew something had to give somewhere.

An Official Diagnosis

Finally in 2017, a doctor listened to me and sent me to a psychologist under the guise of getting more stress management skills. This psychologist diagnosed me with GAD and suggested that I might be autistic, although she was not qualified to diagnose adults. I learned many new coping skills and was relieved to hear someone else share my opinion, but the imposter syndrome was still there: Are we sure I am autistic? What if I am not? Then what is wrong with me? By this time I was comfortable self-identifying as autistic but was still desperate to hide it, just in case I was wrong, and I was afraid of what others would think of me if they knew. It would take a few more years before I could start to accept myself as not broken.

The skills I learned to cope with anxiety did help, but they still failed to solve things entirely. My therapist also introduced me to some autism-coping tools like noise-canceling headphones and a weighted blanket—both felt like wonderful relief. Still, this did not entirely solve my problem at work. For example, some days I would have classes in the morning and still be teaching classes in the evenings. I would become fatigued and then get headaches and sometimes had to vomit in the bathroom between classes to cope. I asked for shorter days, but ashamed to mention my deficiencies, I expressed it as a want, and things really did not change. To facilitate change I would have to share something more concrete with someone and probably get an official diagnosis.

Pursuing a diagnosis when fighting autistic burnout yet still trying to mask as normal was extremely difficult. First, insurance would not cover it, so this would be entirely out-of-pocket—and diagnoses are not cheap. Second, psychologists, psychiatrists, therapists . . . everywhere I turned I kept getting denied and told they only dealt with children or those under 21. I guess, since I had survived this long being "broken," fixing me really was not a priority.

The COVID-19 pandemic brought two positives into my life. First, the isolation from others was a much-needed recovery time. Working from home, I was able to control my environment and the times I worked. I no longer had to deal with people and social expectations. It became clear to me how sensory unfriendly I had found my previous environments. Second, I also found a psychologist willing to diagnose me. In 2020 I finally received an official autism diagnosis. This was very validating and an extreme relief. At last, I could set the imposter syndrome to rest; I was never broken, just different. I also started learning about my other co-occurring conditions during this time.

Disclosing to Others

Deciding to disclose my autism to others was an intimidating idea, but I would probably never get the help I needed otherwise. Unfortunately, one of my first attempts to disclose involved asking for official accommodations, which were denied. The process was stressful, and I left feeling invalidated as well as unsuccessful and inadequate. Luckily, I disclosed to a few others, and most reactions ranged from curious to positive. Some people were willing to help me in a less formal capacity. Some people thought I was brave. Some people wanted to know more about neurodiversity.

I started to consider: Should I stop hiding my autism and other mental health issues? I was tired of constantly trying to fit in, and it really was not working. Was I truly strong enough to withstand any of the different types of reactions I would get—positive and negative? How many others were out there struggling alone and invisible?

At the end of the fall 2021 semester, a student approached me and apologized for not doing well in my class. He said he suffered from GAD. He was sure it was a great class, but he just could not cope. He wanted me to know his failure was not my fault; I could see the shame in his eyes and how much it was costing him to tell me. This event still fills me with anger. Here is an individual whom we could possibly have helped if he had approached me sooner. He did not come forward because of the shame and stigma surrounding his condition.

This event gave me pause. I thought back through the years and realized that, unfortunately, this was not an isolated incident. Many other students out there were struggling with neurodiversity and mental health conditions. I wondered if getting accommodations for these students would be as challenging as my own experience. The stigma and attitudes associated with these conditions are wrong. Society bears some of the responsibility for creating and perpetuating this toxic environment, and we must do better! How can we make neurodivergent individuals feel safe and included and get them the support they need?

How can I make a difference? I want to show that you can be neurodiverse or have mental health issues and still be successful. I want people to be aware that I (and others like me) may be different, but we are not less. There may be challenges, but there are also strengths associated with autism and other neurodiverse conditions.

My Advocacy Begins

I began to consider what positive actions we could take in higher education to improve the situation. I started reading and researching neurodiversity in adults and higher education. I was disappointed at the lack of effort put forth here. These conditions are still too often considered childhood conditions, but neurodivergent children become neurodivergent adults.

I started to take small actions myself. I voiced how noisy and bothersome overhead lights could be, bringing awareness to sensory differences; I started to use my fidgets out in the open; I started sharing parts of my story with students and colleagues across the college. I realized my need for routine and structure was an autistic strength that shone through as organization in my classes. I leaned into universal design and trauma-informed teaching and allowed students to use fidgets in the classroom.

Thankfully, sharing my own neurodiverse perspective has been largely welcomed by my colleagues and students. One of my students with OCD in the fall 2022 semester tearily claimed that nobody had ever really understood him before. Another young woman remarked on how great it was to be able to know someone who shared her struggles. I realized that our neurodivergent students must be able to see themselves among the staff, and the only way this can happen is for staff to understand and be willing to share. I can do that! That can be my way of combating the stigma.

We need to normalize neurodivergence and mental health. This can start with me and my actions in the classroom, but efforts need to expand beyond that. What is already happening that is positive regarding neurodiversity? What could we be doing that we are not doing? I do not know. This is where I am focusing my research and practices. It is now time to gather allies and take actions to promote acceptance and inclusion. My goal is to continue learning about neurodiversity and mental health; to be an advocate for the equity and inclusion of neurodiverse people, specifically in the college environment.

I am still learning about myself and my diagnosis, and how to help others. Mental health is not my area of expertise, but I can speak from my experiences, and I have learned my experiences have value. Too few neurodiverse voices in higher education are challenging the stigmas around these conditions. I aim to be one of these voices.

FOURTEEN

Born Under a Bad Sign

An African American Experience in Higher Education

KYLE YOUNGER

CONFUSED, I SAT very still and thought about what my former guidance counselor had just asked me: "How did you get into this school?" Though I had graduated with a 3.8 GPA, my attendance at this school was puzzling to her. In some ways it was puzzling to me as well. I was existing, sometimes struggling, and sometimes flourishing in the atmosphere of higher education that clearly was not designed for me to succeed. I felt like Bigger Thomas in Richard Wright's (2008) *Native Son* when he said, "The thing to do was to act just like others acted, live like they lived, and while they were not looking, do what you wanted." I had tried that though, and it did not work. I was still different from my peers. Thankfully, I did not end up like Bigger Thomas, though I knew too many who did.

I was different not only from my white peers but also from my Black ones. In time I would learn exactly why. In the early 2000s, I was diagnosed with bipolar II and generalized anxiety disorder and decided not to disclose this to my employers or peers. The major feature of my diagnosis is depression marked by episodes of hypomania. Due to existing stressors related to being African American in mostly white-dominated spaces, I did not want leadership and the dominant culture of academia to have additional reasons to disqualify or discredit my work, efforts, or qualifications. To explore this phenomenon, I have sought out scholarly literature related to the topic and statistical evidence and combined these elements with my own personal journey as an African American man employed in higher education.

Mental Health and Stigma

Getting diagnosed with a mood disorder is not easy for a moody and odd Black kid navigating on the fringes. Mental health stigma manifests when individuals or groups have negative thoughts and beliefs related to mental illness or mental health treatment (DeFreitas et al. 2018, 49). Stigma is associated with negative outcomes including but not limited to discrimination, reduced usage of mental health services, and poor mental health outcomes (49). When stigma is strong, individuals will avoid treatment and suffer in silence until the disorder approaches levels of incapacitation (49). As an African American man in academia, I was already somewhat of an anomaly. Since I was young, it seemed that the structures in which I was navigating were expecting me to fail or somehow be less. If I were to reveal my mental health status as an African American in higher education, I would be fulfilling that societal perspective.

I made the decision, therefore, to not divulge my struggles with mental illness. I did not want and do not want to be a stereotype. Insights from critical race theory (CRT) sensitized me to the concept of structural determinism (Delgado and Stefancic 2013; Tsai 2021). Of all the concepts in CRT, structural determinism was the most elusive. When I understood, it made me want to stay one step ahead. I recognized how things can seem predetermined when I noticed the way mental illness could limit possibilities for me even when decent people want to be inclusive and supportive. If there is systemic racism, maybe we are admirable for overcoming adversity, but while we overcome adversity, organizations need people who are not damaged or distracted. If they want to take on some Black people despite how damaged we might be, then they can check that box without going so far as to include a Black man with mental illness.

Even without the added aspect of being a person of color, mental illness carries with it many problematic stigmas. Common stigmas related to mental illness are that sufferers are dangerous, that they will not recover, and that their mental illness is their own fault (DeFreitas et al. 2018, 49). The most painful part of the notion that it is their own "fault" is the way they subjectively may begin to feel it is indeed their fault if they are stigmatized because of their behavior and speech. Is nothing our fault? Where is the line between what is and is not the fault of someone experiencing an interplay of mental health challenges and other adversity?

When stigma is present, those with mental health struggles have low employment rates, poor/unsafe housing, and a reduction in mental health care (DeFreitas et al. 2018, 49). Self-medication through alcohol demonstrated itself as an almost expected phenomenon for someone like me who made the initial choice not to receive mental health care. It was easier to have a couple of shots of vodka before going to work than to call in sick because I needed a mental health day to take care of myself. How would I explain to my boss or colleagues that I was sick, when physically I was just fine?

When mental health stigma is compounded with the normalcy of anti-Blackness in the United States, a double jeopardy manifests. Within this framework I asked myself whether or not I would be more inclined to speak among my peers about my mental illness if I were not Black. Already, I often find myself code-switching to fit in with the dominant culture, which in and of itself can become draining. Nearly every day after work, I would come home and need at least an hour to decompress from the depression I was experiencing and the microaggressions that were all too prevalent. Accepting that anti-Blackness is a real phenomenon is part of coping with the microaggressions, even when I am being gaslit or told that I am making a "big deal" out of my experience. For this reason it is important to have a strong support system outside the institution. Through self-reflection I have determined that mental health stigma, even if removed from the African American experience, is sufficiently present in my academic experience that I likely would make the same decision again not to disclose my personal struggles to my employer and peers. On the other hand, without the added stressors of the African American experience in higher education, I would be more likely to do so. The microaggressions related to stigmas of both Black academics and mental health are both very strong alone and even stronger when paired together.

Mental Health in Academia

Mental health problems have an impact on the general population in a statistically significant capacity. Quijada (2021) puts the number at 19.1%, which means that 1 in 5 individuals suffers from mental illness. Ward et al. (2013) estimated that 57.5 million American adults suffer from mental illness. Among academics the number is estimated to be higher. Morrish (2019) concluded that rises in mental health struggles of 50% to 316% among academics has been the norm in recent years. The University of Kent, for example, has had a 424% rise in occupational health referrals, and Keele University was at a 344% increase (Morrish 2019). The nature of work in academia can be stressful, thereby contributing to the phenomenon (Quijada 2021). Contributing factors include but are not limited to excessive workloads, audit metrics, contracts, tenure, and performance management elements (Morrish 2019). Morrish described higher education as an "anxiety machine" (1).

Being a first-generation college student from a lower-middle-class family in the predominantly Black city of Newark, New Jersey, presented few mentors or examples at home or from the neighborhood of what a Black academic would look like. All I knew was that I wanted to get out of my neighborhood and that education was the key to achieving this. Periods of mania aided me in finishing my degree, and by the completion of my first masters, I ended up with my first job in higher education as an adjunct professor. It is important to note that academics who identify their work as more demanding, who perceive greater rewards, and who are less overcommitted a lower measure of well-being across all measures (Kinman 2016). Students working toward challenging advanced degrees have also recorded high rates of mental health struggles (Beddoes and Danowitz 2022). Though institutions of higher learning are generally progressive and embrace diversity, stigma still exists for those professionals working in the field and struggling with mental illness (Quijada 2021). Individuals already suffering from mental health struggles who enter the academic world find themselves in a job likely to increase that struggle (Quijada 2021). This was the case for me as I eventually worked toward earning my doctorate.

As an African American instructor in higher education, I discovered that students seemed enthusiastic about having a Black man as a professor. For some students, it was their first experience with having a Black male teacher of any kind. While this was my experience working at a junior college, by the time I moved on to adjunct teaching at predominantly white institutions, I found I was often met with surprised looks. I recall that during one student's presentation, Black people were referred to as "colored." When the student evaluations came in at the end of the semester, one student commented, "How is someone who speaks Ebonics teaching at this school?" In short, racism was prevalent. Even when I was embraced, it was more as a mascot than as an equal to my white peers. On the other end of the spectrum, one African American student stated that it was good "to see one of us teaching" at the school. Even under supportive conditions, it was framed as an "us" and "them" scenario rather than one of learning and the advancement of human beings.

Mental Health and African Americans

While there are some mixed results related to mental health propensity and the African American experience, the bulk of the data suggest that though African Americans make up only 12% of the U.S. population, they make up 18.7% of those impacted by mental illness (Ward et al. 2013, 185). Some studies have suggested that ethnic minorities may have higher levels of stigma than European Americans (DeFreitas et al. 2018, 49). When compared to Caucasians, mentally ill African Americans have more chronic diseases, higher rates of disability, higher rates of inpatient service use, more barriers to seeking treatment, and lower rates of outpatient care (Ward et al. 2013, 185). Though research has increased related to African Americans and mental illness, there are currently gaps related to gender and age differences among this demographic (185). Despite this, stigma has been identified as a significant barrier to mental health service usage among African Americans (Masuda et al. 2012). Mental health stigma among minorities has been identified as primarily stemming from a lack of knowledge/awareness about the reality of mental illness (DeFreitas et al. 2018, 49). A study conducted by Ward and Heidrich (2009) sheds light on the beliefs of African American women regarding the causes and consequences of mental illness (Ward and Heidrich 2009). It found that these women perceived mental illness as a complex interplay of family-related stress, social stress due to racism, and a cyclical nature. Furthermore, the study pointed out that seeking treatment was seen as a way to exert some control over these serious consequences.

Reflecting on this research, I find that the impact of social stress due to racism is an ever-present reality, even when it may not be overt. There is an unfortunate tendency for some individuals to assume that people of color, like myself, are "diversity hires," which undermines our hard work, qualifications, and accomplishments. This constant scrutiny and doubt often create a feeling that we must prove ourselves constantly to gain acceptance and legitimacy in academic and professional settings. The academic environment, though designed to foster learning and growth, often fails to be affirming for individuals from diverse backgrounds. Instead it tends to reinforce the norms and values of the dominant culture, making it challenging to fully embrace one's identity without feeling the need to conform. The emotional toll of these experiences can be overwhelming, leading to feelings of exhaustion and disillusionment when it seems like little progress is being made to change the prevailing dynamic. In such an environment, it is easy to feel like you are just going through the motions to earn a paycheck rather than truly thriving and contributing to your field of study.

While a great deal of literature, some of which I have cited in this discourse, has identified a resistance among people of color to seeking mental health services, less has focused on the journey for those people of color who have elected to receive help. This creates another element that I believe compounds the existing disparity. For me, it was difficult finding a therapist who was a Black man, which is where my comfort level was at for wanting to disclose my personal struggles. Mental health is a white-dominated profession, and based on my experience of the aforementioned microaggressions, I was concerned that I would lack the therapeutic bond I needed if I was working with someone who could not draw upon similar experiential references. While watching peers work with African American students, I often viewed instances of paternalism and infantilization of the students with whom they worked. I feared this phenomenon could potentially hinder the quality of help I sought to receive.

I did not believe my situation was unique, and as an academic I sought out research related to this perception. Evidence backed my own trepidation. Goode-Cross and Grim (2016) concluded that Black clients frequently preferred working with mental health providers of African descent. A myriad of reasons were evidenced for this, including but not limited to an innate connection to other Black people, a result of cultural mistrust embedded within the African American identity and evidence of clients' advanced racial identity status (Goode-Cross and Grim 2016). These factors are more likely a blend of cultural, philosophical, and epistemological elements. The situation goes both ways as additional evidence suggests that Black therapists feel they have a sense of solidarity with Black clients that better helps them understand the context of their struggles, thereby creating faster therapeutic connections.

While there is clearly a connection between African American therapists and African American clients, with clients of color wanting to work with people who better understand their experience, there is a shortage of mental health professionals who meet this criterion. Specifically, only 4.1% of therapists in the United States are Black, and among therapists in general, women make up 70% (Zauderer 2023). Personally, for this reason I was unable to find an African American therapist, but my understanding of mental struggles drove me to continue seeking a professional with whom I could form a sufficient therapeutic bond. My current therapist is not African American, but he truthfully disclosed that his wife was. This led me to question how many African Americans are not obtaining mental health services because of a lack of therapists who are like them.

Mental Health and African Americans in Academia

Few studies specifically relate to African American staff at institutions of higher learning and mental health struggles. On a personal level, the microaggressions tax my mental health. They cause anger, frustration, sadness, and even self-doubt. Chronic emotional distress, I have found, triggers mental health episodes. How do I tell my white boss that I am taking a mental health day because of racism and a bipolar diagnosis? Exploring this further, Mulzac concluded that individuals of color in academia must expend a great deal of effort to excel in an environment with such a degree of chronic interpersonal and institutional racism that their humanity is often overlooked (Mulzac 2022).

Challenges related to teaching, researching, publishing, mentoring, and administrating while also dealing with tension related to race are compounding (Mulzac 2022). In general, African American faculty constitute a small number at most institutions but have unique physical, psychological, emotional, spiritual, social, and legal struggles related to the experience (Alexander and Moore 2008). In these environments, African American faculty can face isolation, exclusion, and cultural taxation that builds on a foundation of the aforementioned climates of stress in academia at large (Mulzac 2022). Even among psychology departments, Whitten (2022) identified the continued presence of a "debilitating stigma of mental illness" in higher education. Whitten, in a personal reflection of his own struggle as a Black faculty member in a psychology department, stressed that living with bipolar disorder prevented colleagues from intervening and providing needed support during crises. The stigmas present raise concerns related to their impact on personal and professional lives. Mental health professional peer opinions have manifested an environment where professionals of African descent rarely share the details of their own mental health struggles (Whitten 2022, 35).

Within this context, I find that taking time off to care for my mental health is paramount for my own well-being as well as my efficacy as a professional. Recently, the heavily spotlighted killings of unarmed Black people like George Floyd and Tyre Nichols were particularly troubling. When these images were replayed constantly, it reminded me that this could have been me or one of my relatives. The additional stress and sadness this caused myself and likely other people of color in similar positions added to my anxiety and mental health struggles. There is a disconnect between current events and their impact on the mental health of African American professionals. Some strides have been made to rectify this. Prior to the George Floyd murder, institutions would not even acknowledge the incident. These days it is common for employees to receive letters from the university president outlining the university's stance and commitment to diversity, equity, and inclusion. As appreciated as it is for these incidents to be acknowledged, it would be even better if there was more recognition of the sadness and stress these events cause for their employees of color.

Conclusions

The intersection of my identity as an African American man with a mental illness has had a profound impact on my higher education experience. I have faced both personal and systemic barriers in my academic and professional journey. Personally, I have had to deal with stereotypes and microaggressions as a Black man with a mental illness, which can create a hostile environment. I see positive dynamics in society as a whole. For example, the commitment to diversity is at an all-time high. There is a general cultural and organizational underpinning that accepts strength in diversity. This is a good start, but where the limitations of a popular organizational buzzword begin and where actual meaningful interventions to promote it properly begin are not universally agreed upon. As an African American man in academia, I do not feel that diversity is fully realized or appreciated, as evidenced by microaggressions, paternalism, and a culture of "otherness." Whenever there is a Black issue, others often reach out to me to speak on behalf of all Black people, or treat me as if I have some secret power that only other Black people can understand. This is obviously problematic and creates a feeling of being "tokenized." Is it my perspective that is valued based on merit or my perspective based on the fact that I was born Black?

Similarly, mental health struggles are more openly discussed and more normalized than perhaps they have ever been in history. This has not been sufficient enough for me to "come out" as suffering from bipolar II and generalized anxiety disorder. As an African American, I am marginalized, and as a person suffering from mental illness, I am also marginalized. To achieve that which diversity and inclusion can be, the first step is honest discourse that requires listening and sharing in a nonjudgmental capacity. In the current environment of "cancel culture" and "wokeness," while the sentiment may be good, the way it comes out in practice can create further division and fear of honest conversation. No one wants to say the "wrong" thing and be ostracized. The entire situation and its complexity are such that it is uncomfortable, and in situations where asking questions is necessary, people stay silent out of fear. I do not speak for all African American men any more than I speak for all academics; speaking and listening, however, seems to me to be a positive way forward toward realizing the benefits of diversity and providing the support needed for all of us.

BONUS CHAPTERS

FIFTEEN

"It's Okay to Be Human" and Other Lessons Learned Under My Desk

KATRINA SWINEHART HELD

THIS PAST ACADEMIC YEAR, I completed my 12th year as an educator. During this time I have taught thousands of students. I have learned how to comfort students having a difficult time. In providing comfort and support, one of my commonly used phrases is "Being a human is hard." I had never applied that phrase to myself when I had a hard time, however. At least not until daily panic attacks under my desk became part of my routine during my first year as a tenure-track faculty member.

The moment I began to believe that I needed to accept my human nature was the day that I came home from work after experiencing two different panic attacks, teaching three lectures, and attending several meetings while functioning on only a few hours of sleep and then deciding I should somehow have the brainpower to tackle a few hours of grading and homework. I felt awful. I was exhausted. I was done. That winter evening, I settled on the couch with a glass of wine and some Kleenex to cry a good cry instead. That is the day I realized I was human. I was a tired human. I was a tired human who needed to do something different. Thankfully, I found my way to therapy to get the help I needed. I want to share the lessons I have learned from my experiences as a neurodivergent doctoral student and faculty member.

My Neurodiversity

Growing up in the Appalachian region of Ohio, mental health was not something we directly addressed or acknowledged during my childhood. Mental health was something I began to pay attention to during my master's degree program at Ohio State University when I was stressed about balancing all of my roles and tasks. My adviser suggested I talk to someone to help me process and manage my stress. Later, during my first year of teaching, a doctor addressed my panic attacks en route to work as "female hysteria," wherein he provided medicine to help with my "intense feelings." It was not until I entered my faculty position, however, that I was finally able to identify a path forward that provided holistic support for my mental health.

During my first year as a tenure-track faculty member, I noticed that I was experiencing fits of panic, often ending with lengthy panic attacks that had me hiding under my desk to conceal my mental health. After weeks of struggling with daily attacks, I acknowledged that I was human, that being human was hard, and that I needed help. I only realized this after a week of little sleep, daily panic attacks, and being nudged by my partner to notice that my physical health was declining.

In February 2019 I located a mental health clinic in town that could address all aspects of my mental health issues. I was provided an appointment with my first psychologist, who utilized tools and the *Diagnostic and Statistical Manual V* to diagnose me. I also visited a neuropsychologist and felt very confident that her observations and suggested plan would be of value to me long-term. This medical team helped to diagnose me with generalized anxiety disorder, bipolar II disorder, and attention deficit hyperactivity disorder (ADHD). I have been lucky to be able to handle these issues using therapy, coaching, and medication. I am cognizant, however, that these challenges influence my choices and experiences daily during my professional work. This is not something I take lightly, and I am mindful of this while entering spaces with students who may also need to manage their mental health in their path forward. This chapter seeks to address the modalities of my professional work during my journey with mental illness.

My Higher Education Positionality

I had the privilege of having a unique position as a doctoral student alongside my tenure-track position for five academic years before I graduated this past summer. Being a student and a faculty member simultaneously provided the opportunity for powerful reflection on my choices. My faculty member role informed how I engaged with the faculty teaching my doctoral courses. My time as a doctoral student with identified neurodiversity was rife with both positive and negative experiences, although these experiences allowed me to understand how to work with students with mental illness and/or neurodiversity in the classroom and as an adviser. Hopefully, these nuggets of knowledge from my own life can provide some enlightenment on your path to supporting students struggling with mental illness, distress, or neurodiversity while completing their education.

Be Kind Whenever Possible. It's Always Possible.—Dalai Lama

Early in my mental health journey, I learned the power of words. In one particularly alarming class session I attended as a student, during a faculty-led discussion numerous students were able to demean or insult the views of others. They did so in calculated, unkind ways to shut down differing viewpoints. The professor did nothing to redirect the conversation, and the negativity spiraled. The two-hour class lagged with more discussion, making it difficult to focus due to my distress until finally, the professor ended class for the day, and I logged off to process the experience. My reflections led me to believe that my views were not valued, my opinion was not respected, and I needed to be more guarded in my engagement within the class discussion space for this course. I felt discouraged and frustrated, as I had been enjoying the course. Future class discussions lost their robust content and variety of thought. Given our fear of being demeaned, what did I not share, or what was not shared by others? We will never know. I felt dejected and dismissed. I finished the class by completing the minimum assignments needed to earn an A and checked out otherwise. I did so to protect my mental health.

Do not let this be your classroom. Inclusive pedagogy dictates that to be equitable, the instructor should set ground rules for class discussions, have a preset cue for students to show you if they are feeling uncomfortable, and know your students so you can tell if they are uncomfortable (this is discussed more later in the chapter). Also, all discussions must be based on the course readings or related literature. By laying out these basic requirements for class discussion or your classroom environment, you will subvert any attempt to stop upholding the tone of collegiality and kindness in that space. Even with the best guidelines, however, at some point you will likely have to step up to enforce these expectations. This sounds easy enough for some but is terrifying for others. In redirecting our class tone and student discourse, addressing the structural features that could make this tough is important.

How can supporting students in this way be tough? To begin, contingent and untenured faculty will systematically feel the need to have all students like them (and their class) so they can get the positive student evaluations needed at the end of the semester to make a case for returning next semester or eventually earning tenure. This systematic way of letting faculty feel this pressure to ensure that the "customers" like the "service" they receive has paralyzed instructors' ability to react and protect the concept of respect in their classrooms. If you are a faculty member who is neurodiverse or experiencing mental illness, you will likely have a heightened reaction to the need to fit in and avoid causing issues. This might lead you to fear the repercussions of taking action to keep an equitable, kind environment. I learned long ago in working with students that how you say things, not always the message itself, determines how feedback is received. As a neurodiverse person, I can purport how I would react to specific feedback, but I have also found that it can bias my understanding of how others could interpret my feedback. I have found that negative feedback sandwiched between positive feedback and a plan to work on the issue often helps the message to be better received. Keep that in mind. Suppose you are particularly concerned about delivering feedback in person. I have found that practicing my feedback in a mirror to view my body language and facial expression is helpful to ensure that I am conveying the tone I want to share with the student.

This need for kindness expands beyond ensuring it in the classroom. As an authority figure to students in various ways, faculty must be mindful of how they communicate with students individually and in groups. Again, practicing in a mirror and creating curated messages that include positive feedback and growth plans for the future are important. I have learned that I often have no idea about the challenges students are facing outside their schoolwork, so I always want to be supportive while delivering difficult feedback. Most recently, I had a student in my office who had missed a few weeks of class and at least one assignment; the student stopped by to let me know that she had lost a few family members to gang violence. She was already distraught about getting caught up on the work and was being hard on herself for having such a difficult time with her loss. This is just one example during my career in which I was so glad that I checked on the student's well-being before even thinking about broaching the subject of her attendance or grade.

Neurodivergent faculty might experience difficulty reading and understanding social cues from students while working through these situations. I have gotten better at reading student behavior the longer I have been in the classroom. Experience is not the only teacher regarding reading cues and body language, however. Asking clarifying questions such as "Can you tell me more about how you are feeling?," or "I believe you might be feeling in [insert your belief] way; could you help me understand if I am on the right track?" By seeking clarification instead of assuming, you will likely make the student feel more comfortable and appreciate your concern. If you experience such difficulties, you might also try sharing that with students at the start of a conversation. You can simply say, "I do not like to assume what you are feeling or conveying with your body language, so I might ask you some clarifying questions if that is okay?" I have seen great tools online that talk about body language and social cues from various cultures; using some tools to help you garner more knowledge in this aspect of student communication might also be helpful. When working with students, just be kind.

It is simple enough. The Dalai Lama was on to something important, but I would tweak the quote slightly: "Be kind whenever possible. It's always possible, so do not make excuses for your actions."

Get to Know Your Students

It is difficult to know whether a student's behavior or emotions are atypical if you have not familiarized yourself with their baseline behaviors and emotions. My colleagues, advisers, and a course instructor who noticed a change in my behavior and emotions helped me decide to seek help. Just the questions "You seem quiet today; is everything okay?" or "How are you really doing?" posed to a student might be a trigger to help them open up to divulge their thoughts. I have found that students, and even myself, need permission to share what we consider "heavy" topics. If students seem hesitant to share, it is important to remind them that it is not required. It is also crucial to let students know that you are there to support them if they ever want to talk. I am amazed at the number of students I have worked with who have few individuals they can talk to during times of distress or stress. Just reaching out to another person can make a tremendous difference.

Additionally, it is important to get to know who your students are; beyond your classroom and their behavior, it can help build a strong bond, which is important for student motivation. If this interests you, explore self-determination theory (SDT), which places relationships with others in a learning environment as one of three components influencing student motivation (Deci et al. 1991). SDT purports that individuals will feel more motivated when their experiences lead them to believe they are able to complete the work (competence), are connected to others in their learning environment (relatedness), and are able to make some decisions for themselves in the learning process (autonomy) (Deci et al. 1991). One of the ways that I accomplish this is to have my students fill out an information sheet each semester. I read them over, note a few pieces of information about each student on my personal attendance sheet, and talk to students about what they shared. These relationships have supported students in getting the resources they need for their college experience, career development, and plans after graduation. Personally, the professors, teachers, colleagues, and friends who identified that I "wasn't acting in my usual way" have allowed me to feel valued and cared for during my experiences. I would credit those check-ins with saving my life during my teen years and young adulthood. You never know what thoughts and plans students have in their brains. Some students may not want to share many personal details, so meet them where they are regarding information about their life outside of class.

University structures can make it difficult to get to know students, especially after we returned to more face-to-face activities on campus after the pandemic. Faculty have an overwhelming number of responsibilities, which causes them to forget things. From personal experience, this is even more true for faculty experiencing neurodiversity or mental illness. I remember to engage in interaction with students by taking an agenda for each class session, reminding myself to talk to at least two students about something important to them before or after each class. My ADHD brain needs that extra reminder and the routine of writing the task down to complete it. I rotate through my class roster throughout the semester abstractly. These engagements can affect student belonging and their sense of having a relationship with you. These campus connections promote student persistence through their degree program.

Another university structure to acknowledge here is the unwritten rhetoric that often leads to biased, unrealistic expectations of our colleagues. At some institutions, female faculty might be expected to take on more "caring" roles within a unit, or comments may be made when you are not overly kind and welcoming to a male colleague at an event. Minority faculty and contract or adjunct faculty might also experience such events. It is important to note that we cannot expect varying levels of kindness from different groups of individuals in our environment. We need to be equitable in the kindness we expect from our colleagues, and expectations of kindness being demonstrated to students must also be equitable.

University structures, especially the heavy faculty workloads, make it difficult for faculty to use their time and energy to engage students.

So find a system for you that works for you. One of my colleagues has created a time each week to meet with students in the campus cafeteria for a meal. They change the meal throughout the semester and allow an open invitation for any student (current or former) to join them. It has been amazing to see this group of students growing to regularly join this "long-table" model of relationship building. You have to find an authentic way to connect with students, so my best advice is just to do "you" and see how your relationships with students change for the better.

Demonstrate Care When You Can

In my classes I greet students individually as they enter the classroom and/or wish them well on their way out. My students at CSU love to tease me, but my favorite closing to a class is to wish the students a "Happy [Day of the Week]! Make good choices." As all educators know, our students face challenges on a daily basis, and sometimes the challenges are compounded by many dark, negative forces. I have worked with students who have had to make difficult choices between loved ones and their education due to addiction, crime, or mental illness in their family. On occasion I have met students who have had to leave school to care for younger siblings after the loss of a family member to gang activity or drug addiction. This often leads to a great deal of depression and anxiety for the student. Trying to stay positive and provide support can make a big difference for them, even if you do not directly see it.

During a recent semester, I had a new encounter with providing care for students. A homesick student had tried different friend groups but could not any she felt connected to, so she desperately wanted to go home. The student had mentioned several times that she just missed her dogs at home and felt she needed that connection to improve her mental health to stay on campus. Against all my training as a former K–12 educator and all my fears about something problematic happening, I brought the student to my home one afternoon to help me take my dogs for a walk and play with them. Immediately, the student started crying. You would have to know my beagle/basset dog, Gary, but he is a natural therapy dog and a top-notch cuddler. On particularly rough days, I have also sobbed while cuddling Gary. Afterward, the student seemed much more light and commented on how much better she felt. Honestly, my dogs also had a wonderful afternoon! On the way back to campus, we got dinner. The student expressed a tremendous amount of gratitude. She will be leaving our campus certain that we care about our students deeply beyond just classroom success. I do not regret opening my home and sharing my pets with this student. Demonstrating care for students can look like many other things, though.

Demonstrating care for students could take any route, as care should be customized to the student or students you are hoping to support. In my example above, sharing a meal and time with my dogs demonstrated kindness. But you could also attend a sporting event, theater production, or other campus event to support students. You could also demonstrate care by bringing snacks to class sessions, providing a list of resources for students, or supporting students when they need to miss class for a mental health day. *Ted Lasso*, an Apple TV show that follows the story of an American football coach who moves to London to coach a professional soccer team, provides exemplary examples of an authority figure demonstrating care for his subordinates. Ted shows his care and affection for each player differently and supports the staff as unique individuals. Ted is known for delivering biscuits to the team owner daily, having small group meetings with the manager and coaching staff to address personal and team issues, and creating special handshakes/greetings with each player. We could all take a lesson from the depths of care Ted demonstrates toward everyone he encounters throughout the show. Ted is also known for giving great advice. My favorite Ted Lasso advice would probably be as follows: "Taking on a challenge is a lot like riding a horse, isn't it? If you're comfortable while you're doing it, you're probably doing it wrong" (*Ted Lasso* 2020).

As a student and faculty member, I found that the level of education you are teaching does not matter; those who are supportive of students might be viewed differently. I have worked in places where those who attended events and demonstrated support for students were applauded and encouraged by administrators. Since my time in higher education, however, I have also heard whispers that those who provide extra care for their students are not likely to be rigorous instructors or are a "pushover" for students. I am not entirely sure that is true from my own experiences. In higher education, where peers vote on promotions and tenure requests and adjunct assignments are controlled by peer department chairs, it can be easy to feed into the system of trying not to draw extra attention to the process you use to develop relationships with students. While this is far from ideal, I am not sure how the academy should address this issue other than to focus on building an institutional environment of acceptance and support over toxic competition and judgment. We must remember that we are all on the same team with shared goals to serve our students.

Be Open to Understanding Student Needs and Experiences

During my doctoral program, I took a class with a faculty member who demanded a meeting upon receiving my ADA accommodation letter. During our meeting to discuss my needs, he said, "I just want you to know I don't believe in ADHD and do not believe you need these extra 'perks.' You need to develop self-discipline, and I don't teach that." Please, please do not do this. All faculty likely might understand why this is a bad idea. I left this meeting in tears, shaking, after an awkward conversation about perks versus legal requirements. This was the worst class of my academic experience as a university student.

Accommodations may come with different requests than ADA accommodation letters, though. Students may also request you work with them to reset due dates for assignments due to a lengthy illness or family emergency. This situation is being considered more frequently based on what we learned from COVID-19. Faculty should attempt to be reasonable when working with students in this regard. Using their best judgment and any policies required by the university or department to guide their decisions is always the best way to move forward. Regardless of the student's needs, I recommend working with students as partners in assessing accommodations and navigating their needs in the learning environment. This is how I have preferred to address accommodations during my entire education career. Students are usually reasonable and just want to learn; let us help them in the ways they need to succeed.

Removing barriers and giving support is the name of the game. In working with students, it is important that you ask questions to ensure you understand the need to provide the support while also understanding the rationale for their requests. It is also okay to set boundaries for what you can provide to the student; just be clear, direct, and consistent. You also need to set clear expectations to let the student know what you need from them moving forward; it is important to be reasonable, clear, and consistent. Working in a partnership with students is about communication to ensure that everyone has the same understanding and is working toward the same goals.

University structure might cause students to not fight for their needs in the classroom, potentially harming their performance. Students often fear the repercussions of pushing back on faculty who might not want to provide legally required needs or other preferences. I have encountered this situation as a student and as a faculty member. Students are often encouraged when I remind them that it is illegal for faculty to ignore their accommodations and modifications from the Office of Student Empowerment. I encourage students to reach out to an advocate to support them in obtaining accommodations or modifications. I often try to help students in navigating getting their needs met in other classes. Not all universities have a unit that provides advocates for students to learn university processes. As a student I found that having another person to help me understand the rules and expectations in a specific situation was helpful. I had an advocate to help me in the situation with the professor who did not want to provide my accommodations. I wish that all universities valued this and offered this support to their students.

Provide Connections to Resources in a General Way

The only positive thing I was able to master during the online class portion of the pandemic was sharing important messages with students. During the first few weeks of the online class, I provided a list of university and community-based supports for different resources: housing, food pantries, childcare, free health clinics, and many more. I anonymously asked students to share other needed resources and added those to the list. By providing everyone with a list, no one had to identify their needs or struggles to gain information. This resource list is still part of my class materials every semester. Students use the resources and get the help they need. Everyone wins.

Resources on my campus still do not provide detailed lists of this nature to the student population. We have a university-planned food pantry truck that comes to campus monthly, and everyone on campus is invited to participate. This does not support the various other needs among students for toiletries, housing, childcare, or access to prepared healthy meals. The systematic supports in place to manage the most common student needs should be replicated to address these other areas. This is especially true for campuses that serve minoritized populations. Another resource that should be readily available is mental health care and the related medications for specific conditions. Our campus has expanded its counseling services to include online therapy to address students' increased need for mental health support. They made this innovative move due to a lack of campus space and student transportation to off-campus sites for services.

Campus leadership must be quick to address student needs and consider new, unconventional ways to obtain the necessary resources for students. They also need to provide widespread communications to the campus community to ensure that everyone knows about these new resources. I have seen instructors place statements in their syllabi, hanging posters on campus, handing out flyers to students, using campus social media, and using student organizations to promote the message. Thinking outside the box to reach students in the spaces and ways they communicate daily is important when wanting to share messages with them.

Conclusion

Rita Pierson (2013), a lifelong educator, shared in her TED Talk that "every kid needs a champion." Yes, even my adult students need a champion too. Regardless of their neurodiversity, background, future plans, and so on, every university student should have the tools to complete their education. Faculty are here to help in various capacities, as are the other staff and administrators on campus. The issue is to help our students get the resources and support they need to be successful. University systems must also address the mental health and neurodiversity of their staff, faculty, and administrators. My mental health could have been addressed sooner if I had known how to navigate the system and understood the severity of my symptoms. Yes, being a human is hard, and clear access to appropriate resources is essential to help ease this challenge. Neurodiversity and mental health challenges do not lessen the value of a person, and the system needs to find ways to demonstrate this better.

Throughout this chapter, I made suggestions that could be applied to students in your classes. Each of us experiencing neurodiversity and mental health challenges is more than our diagnosis. I wish I had felt more comfortable supporting students with their mental health sooner. I am grateful to be here to remind students that being human is difficult, and everyone must practice self-kindness. I am also thankful to share resources with students and support them to complete their education. I am grateful I got the help I needed to keep serving as a support for my students. Being human is hard, but it gets better when you have a strong support team. I have also learned that I am a better supporter and champion when caring for my own mental and physical health. I approach each student and course with the mindset of being the faculty member I needed as an undergraduate student. So remember, "being human is hard"; just be kind to yourself and others along the way.

SIXTEEN

Coda

Professionalism as Ableism

LEE SKALLERUP BESSETTE

IN HER FOREWORD to this collection, Katie Rose Guest Pryal lays plain the catch-22 that neurodivergent employees in higher education face: "If you have been subject to discrimination these days, then you know it is not about what people say out loud. It is about what people do not say; how they talk *around* what they mean." The examples she gives to illustrate this can all be described as "unprofessional behavior," an accusation I am sure every single neurodivergent employee, inside or outside higher education, has experienced.

This collection's opening essay by Catherine J. Denial examines the "platonic ideal" historian, our internalized vision of what a professor should look like:

> A comfortably affluent, older, white, cisgender man who works diligently in an office crammed with books. His office is often illuminated by shafts of sunlight that spill in through large picture windows, and his every movement causes dust motes to dance. Sometimes, if a historian, this professor ventures out to the archives. There he examines letters, diaries, account books, and newspapers, perhaps indulging in a little paleography in order to discover new secrets. The reading room in which he works is always outfitted with wooden shelves and tables and trim, and

it is peaceful and perfectly quiet. We are rarely granted a peek into the interiority of that professor's mind, but nothing about the professor suggests turmoil. The professor thrives on solitude and quiet and whatever deep thoughts he is thinking about the past.

This is, to put it another way, what a *professional* in higher education looks like. It is a powerful image to open the collection with because in our own ways, each contributor transgresses this "norm," this definition of professionalism. It is so embedded in our imaginations that it drove Jorden Cummings to depression because she was never going to be "Brian," an idealized professor whose description matches the one Denial provided. Cummings adds: "Brian firmly believes in publish or perish. There is not a project or a grant he will pass up. He believes that working evenings and weekends is required for academic success and that anyone who cannot do so is weak. He does not understand why anyone would not sacrifice everything for an academic career."

All the masks in part 1 were in place so we could pass as professionals within our respective careers. Jim Luke contextualizes the masking to remain professional as an added burden to neurodivergent faculty and staff: "Everybody works to present and maintain a professional identity or academic persona. But, for neurodivergent faculty, it takes more to get and stay 'in character.' . . . We are all playing a role, a part, in this production we call higher education. The difference is that neurodivergent faculty experience a heavier burden of time, effort, energy, and emotion to play our roles in the way our institutions demand."

Professionalism is just our society's acceptable way of saying ageism, sexism, racism, sizeism, and, in the context of this collection, ableism. Being labeled "unprofessional" is not discrimination, even when we know it is. How many neurotypical readers found yourselves thinking, at some point in reading these stories, how unprofessional of them? Did you catch yourself? Did you question why you had that reaction? If you did not, would you have had that reaction if you had not known the backstory, the circumstances of the person? Reflect on how empathy for the individual might have overridden your gut reaction. Think of Shannan Palma's story about asking questions and taking notes, coping (not even masking!) strategies met with hostility. But go back and reread her story; who were the ones truly being unprofessional, Palma or her colleagues or the entire institution? But Palma realized something in declining an exit interview—it would never have mattered because she had been identified as the problem, as being the unprofessional one. Robert Perret shares a similar story of institutions acting unprofessional while labeling him as the issue: "I tried for years to make the situation better, through the ombuds office, human resources, and even the Office for Civil Rights. I did everything I was supposed to do, again, and it was turned against me, again. After 15 years I have finally learned that I cannot benefit from the system, navigate the system, or even coexist with the system. I certainly cannot beat the system. In the end my only avenue of appeal to the social network of academia was to unfollow."

We, the editors, struggled with what the takeaway should be in order for neurotypical readers of this book, those in positions of relative power or privilege within academia, to create a more inclusive workplace, and that advice is to reevaluate your internalized definition of "professionalism." Is it really about the actual work people are doing, or is it about how people are *perceived* while doing the work? In the introduction to my collection, *Affective Labor and Alt-Ac Careers* (University Press of Kansas, 2022), I relay an anecdote about how, after a positive job review, I was still berated by my then-supervisor for not "behaving like staff" and transgressing unspoken professional norms despite doing objectively good work. How many neurodivergent faculty and staff in higher education have had a similar thing happen to them—poor job reviews despite good work due to issues around professionalism or good reviews but no promotions because of "fit" or (again) issues around professionalism or leadership qualities? Ronnie K. Stephens was denied promotion because "Despite meeting and exceeding every marker for promotion, the vice president elected not to advance my application to the board. Her reasoning: I had not distinguished myself as an asset to the college on the basis that I did not have a strong presence at social functions or broad professional relationships with my colleagues." Stephens struggles with social interaction with his peers due to a neurodivergent condition and is held to an unwritten ableism standard of professionalism.

Professionalism has become the catchall reason for dismissing and marginalizing people who do good work outside our society's norms, or could do good work if they were allowed to work in ways labeled "unprofessional." So the question becomes for the neurotypical: How will you react to and then support your colleagues if and when the mask comes off? Or as I put it toward the end of my essay: "I am not sure anyone is ready for a chorus of us revealing who we really are and demanding what we need to feel like we belong."

Professionalism is a value rarely clearly defined within higher education, the ultimate hidden curriculum for employees, and unevenly applied at that. Take the time to have the conversation within your unit to clearly define what "professionalism" means to everyone and then push it forward to discuss all the ways in which it is doing harm. Our institutions are structured around ableism, but this undefined space of "professionalism" is where individuals, units, and leaders can push back. Make the standard something else, or erase it all together. This is something that we can all control.

Abrams, Zara. 2020. "A Crunch at College Counseling Centers." *Monitor of Psychology* 51, no. 6. https://www.apa.org/monitor/2020/09/crunch-college -counseling.

Alexander, Rudolph, and Sharon E. Moore. 2008. "The Benefits, Challenges, and Strategies of African American Faculty Teaching at Predominantly White Institutions." *Journal of African American Studies* 12:4–18.

American Psychological Association. 2021. "Mental Illness and Violence: Debunking Myths, Addressing Realities." *CE Corner.* https://www.apa.org /monitor/2021/04/ce-mental-illness.

Anderson, Greta. 2020a. "Mental Health Needs Rise with Pandemic." *Inside Higher Ed*, September 10. https://www.insidehighered.com/news/2020/09/11 /students-great-need-mental-health-support-during-pandemic.

Anderson, Greta. 2020b. "A Shared Responsibility." *Inside Higher Ed*, February 19. https://www.insidehighered.com/news/2020/02/20/no-shows-burden -counseling-center-resources.

Beddoes, Kacey, and Andrew Danowitz. 2022. "In Their Own Words: How Aspects of Engineering Education Undermine Students' Mental Health." Paper presented at the 2022 American Society for Engineering Education Annual Conference and Exposition, June 26–29, Minneapolis.

Bessette, Lee Skallerup. 2011. "New CRW Summer Feature: Bad Female Academic." *College Ready Writing* (blog), May 23. http://crwarchive.readywriting .org/higher-education/new-crw-summer-feature-bad-female-academic/.

Bessette, Lee Skallerup. 2012. "Becoming a Cliché." *Inside Higher Ed, University of Venus* (blog). https://www.insidehighered.com/blogs/university-venus /becoming-clich%C3%A9.

Bira, Lindsay, and Teresa M. Evans. 2019. "Mental Health in Academia: An Invisible Crisis." *Physiology News Magazine*, no. 115 (Summer). https://www .physoc.org/magazine-articles/mental-health-in-academia-an-invisible-crisis/.

Bonomi, Amy, Emily Nichols, Rebecca Kammes, and Troye Green. 2018. "Sexual Violence and Intimate Partner Violence in College Women with a Mental Health and/or Behavior Disability." *Journal of Women's Health* 27, no. 3: 359–368. https://doi.org/10.1089/jwh.2016.6279.

Brookfield, Stephen D. 2017. *Becoming a Critically Reflective Teacher.* 2nd ed. Jossey-Bass.

Cantor, David, Bonnie Fisher, Susan Chibnall, Shauna Harps, Reanne Townsend, Gail Thomas, Hyunshik Lee, Vanessa Kranz, Randy Herbison, and Kristin

Madden. 2019. "Report on the AAU Campus Climate Survey on Sexual Assault and Misconduct." Campus Climate Survey. Texas A&M University. https://titleix.tamu.edu/wp-content/uploads/2019/10/TAMU_Climate SurveyandAppendices_2019.pdf.

Cassidy, Frederick, Eileen P. Ahearn, and Bernard J. Carroll. 2001. "Substance Abuse in Bipolar Disorder." *Bipolar Disorders* 3, no. 4: 181–188. https://doi .org/10.1034/j.1399-5618.2001.30403.x.

Cech, Erin A., and Tom J. Waidzunas. 2021. "Systemic Inequalities for LGBTQ Professionals in STEM." *Science Advances* 7, no. 3: eabe0933. https://doi.org /10.1126/sciadv.abe0933.

Chen, Jieru, Mikel L. Walters, Leah K. Gilbert, and Nimesh Patel. 2020. "Sexual Violence, Stalking, and Intimate Partner Violence by Sexual Orientation, United States." *Psychology of Violence* 10, no. 1: 110–119. https://doi.org/10 .1037/vio0000252.

Cook, Benjamin Lê, Nhi-Ha Trinh, Zhihui Li, Sherry Shu-Yeu Hou, and Ana M. Progovac. 2017. "Trends in Racial-Ethnic Disparities in Access to Mental Health Care, 2004–2012." *Psychiatric Services* 68, no. 1: 9–16. https://doi .org/10.1176/appi.ps.201500453.

Copland, Christina. 2018. "Making Historians in the Archives." *AHA Today*, May 14. https://www.historians.org/research-and-publications/perspectives -on-history/may-2018/making-historians-in-the-archive.

Deci, Edward L., Robert J. Vallerand, Luc G. Pelletier, and Richard M. Ryan. 1991. "Motivation and Education: The Self-Determination Perspective." *Educational Psychologist* 26, no. 3–4: 325–346. doi:10.1080/00461520.1991.9653137.

DeFreitas, Stacie Craft, Travis Crone, Martha DeLeon, and Anna Ajayi. 2018. "Perceived and Personal Mental Health Stigma in Latino and African American College Students." *Frontiers in Public Health* 6:49.

Delgado, Richard, and Jean Stefancic, eds. 2013. *Critical Race Theory: The Cutting Edge*. Temple University Press.

Denial, Catherine. 2018. *For Those of Us Who Do Not Love the Archives* (blog). https://catherinedenial.org/blog/uncategorized/for-those-of-us-who-do -not-love-the-archives/.

Deo, Meera E. 2022. "Pandemic Pressures on Faculty." *University of Pennsylvania Law Review Online* 170, no. 1: 127–146.

Dolan, Vera L. B. 2023. "'. . . But If You Tell Anyone, I'll Deny We Ever Met': The Experiences of Academics with Invisible Disabilities in the Neoliberal University." *International Journal of Qualitative Studies in Education* 36, no. 4: 689–706.

EEOC (U.S. Equal Employment Opportunity Commission). 2002. "Enforcement Guidance on Reasonable Accommodation and Undue Hardship under the ADA." October 17. https://www.eeoc.gov/laws/guidance/enforcement -guidance-reasonable-accommodation-and-undue-hardship-under-ada.

Evans, Teresa M., Lindsay Bira, Jazmin Beltran Gastelum, L. Todd Weiss, and Nathan L. Vanderford. 2018. "Evidence for a Mental Health Crisis in

Graduate Education." *Nature Biotechnology* 36, no. 3: 282–284. https://doi
.org/10.1038/nbt.4089.

Fitzpatrick, Kathleen. 2021. *Generous Thinking: A Radical Approach to Saving
the University*. Johns Hopkins University Press.

Golden, Shelley D., and Jo Anne L. Earp. 2012. "Social Ecological Approaches
to Individuals and Their Contexts: Twenty Years of Health Education and
Behavior Health Promotion Interventions." *Health Education and Behavior*
39, no. 3: 364–372. https://doi.org/10.1177/1090198111418634.

Goode-Cross, David T., and Karen Ann Grim. 2016. "'An Unspoken Level of
Comfort': Black Therapists' Experiences Working with Black Clients."
Journal of Black Psychology 42, no. 1: 29–53.

Gordon, Darcy. 2022. "Inclusive Teaching Module." Massachusetts Institute of
Technology: MIT OpenCourseWare. Creative Commons BY-NC-SA. https://
ocw.mit.edu/courses/res-7-009-7-int-inclusive-teaching-module-fall-2022.

Gray, Peter. 2015. "Declining Student Resilience: A Serious Problem for
Colleges." *Psychology Today*, September 22. https://www.psychologytoday
.com/us/blog/freedom-learn/201509/declining-student-resilience-serious
-problem-colleges.

Hayes, Steven C., and Jennifer Gregg. 2001. "Functional Contextualism and the
Self." In *Self-Relations in the Psychotherapy Process*, edited by J. Christopher
Muran, 291–311. American Psychological Association. https://doi.org/10.1037
/10391-012.

Hayes, Steven C., Kirk D. Strosahl, and Kelly G. Wilson. 2016. *Acceptance and
Commitment Therapy: The Process and Practice of Mindful Change*. 2nd ed.
Guilford.

Hill, Leah A. 2018. "Disturbing Disparities: Black Girls and the School-to-
Prison Pipeline." *Fordham Law Review Online* 87:58–63.

Hoben, John, and Jackie Hesson. 2021. "Invisible Lives: Using Autoethnogra-
phy to Explore the Experiences of Academics Living with Attention Deficit
Hyperactivity Disorder (ADHD)." *New Horizons in Adult Education and
Human Resource Development* 33, no. 1: 37–50.

Hoots, Brooke E., Jingjing Li, Marci Feldman Hertz, Marissa B. Esser, Adriana
Rico, Evelyn Y. Zavala, and Christopher M. Jones. 2023. "Alcohol and Other
Substance Use before and during the COVID-19 Pandemic among High
School Students—Youth Risk Behavior Survey, United States, 2021."
Morbidity and Mortality Weekly Report Supplements 72, no. 1: 84–92.
http://dx.doi.org/10.15585/mmwr.su7201a10.

Hoover, Elizabeth. n.d. "The Archive Is All in Present Tense." Elizabeth Hoover
Ink (website). http://www.ehooverink.com/narrative-present.html.

Housel, Teresa Heinz. 2023. "The Perfect Storm of Mental Health Issues in
Academia and the Need for Critical Research and Policies." In *Mental
Health among Higher Education Faculty, Administrators, and Graduate
Students: A Critical Perspective*, edited by Teresa Heinz Housel, 3–33.
Lexington Books.

Irish, Bradley J. 2023. "How to Make Room for Neurodivergent Professors." *Chronicle of Higher Education*, March 2. https://www.chronicle.com/article/how-to-make-room-for-neurodivergent-professors.

Johns Hopkins Medicine. 2024. "Mental Health Disorder Statistics." https://www.hopkinsmedicine.org/health/wellness-and-prevention/mental-health-disorder-statistics.

Johnson, Adam P., and Rebecca J. Lester. 2021. "Mental Health in Academia: Hacks for Cultivating and Sustaining Wellbeing." *American Journal of Human Biology* 34, no. S1: e23664.

Khiron Clinics. 2021. "Trauma and Neurodiversity—Understanding the Struggle and Meeting the Needs." *Khiron Clinics* (blog). September 15. https://khironclinics.com/blog/trauma-and-neurodiversity/.

Kinman, Gail. 2016. "Effort-Reward Imbalance and Overcommitment in UK Academics: Implications for Mental Health, Satisfaction and Retention." *Journal of Higher Education Policy and Management* 38, no. 5: 504–518.

Knights, D., and C. A. Clarke. 2014. "It's a Bittersweet Symphony, This Life: Fragile Academic Selves and Insecure Identities at Work." *Organization Studies* 35, no. 3: 335–357.

Lambe, Ariel Mae. 2022. "Seeing Madness in the Archives." *American Historical Review* 127, no. 3: 1384.

Levi, Merry Kalingel, et al. 2023. "'Feeling Unwanted, When Nobody Wants You Around': Perceptions of Social Pain among People with Autism." *American Journal of Occupational Therapy* 77, no. 2. https://doi.org/10.5014/ajot.2023.050061.

Luke, Jim. 2019. "Accessible Lessons at Sea." *EconProph* (blog), March 16. https://econproph.com/2019/03/16/accessible-lessons-at-sea/.

Masuda, Akihiko, Page L. Anderson, and Joshua Edmonds. 2012. "Help-Seeking Attitudes, Mental Health Stigma, and Self-Concealment among African American College Students." *Journal of Black Studies* 43, no. 7: 773–786.

Mellifont, Damian. 2023. "Ableist Ivory Towers: A Narrative Review Informing about the Lived Experiences of Neurodivergent Staff in Contemporary Higher Education." *Disability and Society* 38, no. 5: 856–886.

Meluch, Andrea L. 2023. "Anxiety in Academia: An Autoethnographic Account." In *Mental Health among Higher Education Faculty, Administrators, and Graduate Students: A Critical Perspective*, edited by Teresa Heinz Housel, 35–51. Lexington Books.

Monroe, Scott M., and Kate L. Harkness. 2005. "Life Stress, the 'Kindling' Hypothesis, and the Recurrence of Depression: Considerations from a Life Stress Perspective." *Psychological Review* 112, no. 2: 417–445. https://doi.org/10.1037/0033-295X.112.2.417.

Morrish, Liz. 2019. *Pressure Vessels: The Epidemic of Poor Mental Health among Higher Education Staff*. Higher Education Policy Institute, 2019.

Morrison, Aimée. 2019. "(Un)Reasonable, (Un)Necessary, and (In)Appropriate." *Biography* 42, no. 3: 693–719.

Mulzac, A. C. 2022. "Preserving the Mental Health of Black and Brown Professors in Academia." In *Promoting Mental Wellness*, edited by A. M. Allen and J. T. Steward. Cambridge University Press.

Neuhaus, Jessamyn. 2019. *Geeky Pedagogy*. West Virginia University Press.

Pettit, Emma. 2016. "Stigma, Stress, and Fear: Faculty Mental-Health Services Fall Short." *Chronicle of Higher Education*, August 4. https://www.chronicle.com/article/stigma-stress-and-fear-faculty-mental-health-services-fall-short/.

Pierson, Rita. 2013. "Every Kid Needs a Champion." YouTube, 7:48. May 3. https://www.youtube.com/watch?v=SFnMTHhKdkw.

Pope-Ruark, Rebecca. 2022. *Unraveling Faculty Burnout: Pathways to Reckoning and Renewal*. Johns Hopkins University Press.

Price, Devon. 2022. *Unmasking Autism: Discovering the New Faces of Neurodiversity*. Harmony Books.

Price, Margaret. 2011. *Mad at School: Rhetorics of Mental Disability and Academic Life*. University of Michigan Press.

Price, Margaret, and Stephanie L. Kerschbaum. 2017. *Promoting Supportive Academic Environments for Faculty with Mental Illnesses: Resource Guide and Suggestions for Practice*. Temple University Collaborative. https://tucollaborative.org/wp-content/uploads/2023/08/Promoting-Supportive-Academic-Environments-for-Faculty-with-Mental-Illnesses-Resource-Guide-and-Suggestions-for-Practice.pdf.

Price, Margaret, Mark S. Salzer, Amber O'Shea, and Stephanie L. Kerschbaum. 2017. "Disclosure of Mental Disability by College and University Faculty: The Negotiation of Accommodations, Supports, and Barriers." *Disability Studies Quarterly* 37, no. 2. https://dsq-sds.org/index.php/dsq/article/view/5487/4653.

Pryal, Katie Rose Guest. 2014. "Disclosure Blues: Should You Tell Colleagues about Your Mental Illness." *Chronicle of Higher Education*, June 13. http://dx.doi.org/10.2139/ssrn.4158926.

Pryal, Katie Rose Guest. 2016. "How the TSA Perpetuates Harmful Mental Health Stigmas." *Establishment*, May 12. https://perma.cc/7E2J-78SC; https://medium.com/the-establishment/how-the-tsa-perpetuates-harmful-mental-health-stigmas-90f531962158.

Pryal, Katie Rose Guest. 2024a. "How Suspicion Feeds Stigma against Neurodivergent People." *Psychology Today*, January 13. https://www.psychologytoday.com/intl/blog/living-neurodivergence/202311/how-suspicion-feeds-stigma-against-neurodivergent-people.

Pryal, Katie Rose Guest. 2024b. "Should You Seek an Adult Diagnosis of Neurodivergence?" *Chronicle of Higher Education*, January 22. https://www.chronicle.com/article/should-you-seek-an-adult-diagnosis-of-neurodivergence.

Pryal, Katie Rose Guest. 2024c. "The Struggles and Strengths of Trauma Disorders." *Psychology Today*, March 10. https://www.psychologytoday.com/intl/blog/living-neurodivergence/202403/the-struggles-and-strengths-of-trauma-disorders.

Quijada, Maria Alejandra. 2021. "My Mental Health Struggle in Academia: What I Wish All Business School Faculty, Students, and Administration Knew." *Journal of Management Education* 45, no. 1: 19–42.

Reyes, Marc. 2019. "Why Do Historians Still Have to Go to the Archives?" *Contingent Magazine*, March 25. https://contingentmagazine.org/2019/03/25/mailbag-march-25-2019/.

Rutter, Michael Patrick, and Steven Mintz. 2019. "Are Today's College Students More Psychologically Fragile than in the Past?" *Inside Higher Ed*, April 26. https://www.insidehighered.com/blogs/higher-ed-gamma/are-today%E2%80%99s-college-students-more-psychologically-fragile-past.

Sabagh, Z., N. C. Hall, and A. Saroyan. 2018. "Antecedents, Correlates and Consequences of Faculty Burnout." *Educational Research* 60, no. 2: 131–156.

Sadulski, Jarrod. 2021. "Higher Education Networking during the COVID-19 Pandemic." *EDGE*. American Public University. https://apuedge.com/higher-education-networking-during-the-covid-19-pandemic/.

Schaberg, Christopher. 2021. *Pedagogy of the Depressed*. Bloomsbury Academic.

Shah, Sejal A. 2019. "Even If You Can't See It: Invisible Disability and Neurodiversity." *Kenyon Review*, January/February. https://kenyonreview.org/kr-online-issue/2019-janfeb/selections/sejal-shah-656342/.

Shaw, Claire. 2013. "Higher Education Networking: Engaging Effectively Online and Off—Live Chat." *Guardian*, April 2. https://www.theguardian.com/higher-education-network/blog/2013/apr/02/higher-education-careers-networking-advice.

Shea, Gerard, and Sebastian Derry. 2019. "Academic Libraries and Autism Spectrum Disorder: What Do We Know?" *Journal of Academic Librarianship* 45, no. 4: 326–331.

Sjunneson, Elsa. 2020. "How to Make a Paper Crane from Rage." In *Disability Visibility: First-Person Stories from the Twenty-First Century*, edited by Alice Wong, 134–140. Vintage Books.

Smith, Jacqueline M., et al. 2022. "Exploring Mental Health and Well-Being among University Faculty Members." *Journal of Psychosocial Nursing* 60, no. 11: 17–26.

Starck, Jordan G., Travis Riddle, Stacey Sinclair, and Natasha Warikoo. 2020. "Teachers Are People Too: Examining the Racial Bias of Teachers Compared to Other American Adults." *Educational Researcher* 49, no. 4: 273–284. https://doi.org/10.3102/0013189X20912758.

Stavraki, Ioanna. 2023. "What Is ADHD Masking? Signs You Are Masking and How to Deal with It." December 19. https://www.simplypsychology.org/adhd-masking.html.

Taylor, Helen, and Martin David Vestergaard. 2022. "Developmental Dyslexia: Disorder or Specialization in Exploration?" *Frontiers in Psychology* 13. https://www.frontiersin.org/articles/10.3389/fpsyg.2022.889245.

Ted Lasso. 2020. "Pilot, Episode 1." Apple TV, 31:00. August 14.

Teeter, Christian. 2020. "Professional Networks within U.S. Higher Education: Avenues to Foster Career and Institutional Success." *Journal of Education and Training Studies* 8, no. 6: 1–6.

Thomason, Timothy C. 2012. "A Week in the Life of a University Professor: Issues of Stress, Workload, and Wellness." *Counseling and Wellness: A Professional Counseling Journal* 3:23–36.

Thomeer, Mieke Beth, Myles D. Moody, and Jenjira Yahirun. 2023. "Racial and Ethnic Disparities in Mental Health and Mental Health Care during the COVID-19 Pandemic." *Journal of Racial and Ethnic Health Disparities* 10, no. 2: 961–976. https://doi.org/10.1007/s40615-022-01284-9.

Tsai, Jennifer. 2021. "Building Structural Empathy to Marshal Critical Education into Compassionate Practice: Evaluation of a Medical School Critical Race Theory Course." *Journal of Law, Medicine and Ethics* 49, no. 2: 211–221.

Tyson, Will, Reginald Lee, Kathryn M. Borman, and Mary Ann Hanson. 2007. "Science, Technology, Engineering, and Mathematics (STEM) Pathways: High School Science and Math Coursework and Postsecondary Degree Attainment." *Journal of Education for Students Placed at Risk* 12, no. 3: 243–270. https://doi.org/10.1080/10824660701601266.

Wapnick, Emilie. 2018. *How to Be Everything*. HarperOne.

Ward, Earlise C., and Susan M. Heidrich. 2009. "African American Women's Beliefs about Mental Illness, Stigma, and Preferred Coping Behaviors." *Research in Nursing and Health* 32, no. 5: 480–492.

Ward, Earlise C., Jacqueline C. Wiltshire, Michelle A. Detry, and Roger L. Brown. 2013. "African American Men and Women's Attitude toward Mental Illness, Perceptions of Stigma, and Preferred Coping Behaviors." *Nursing Research* 62, no. 3: 185–194.

Whitten, Lisa. 2022. "Stigma Matters: An African American Psychology Professor Comes out of the Mental Illness Closet." *Psychological Services* 19, no. 1: 35.

Williams, Simon. 2019. "2019 Postgraduate Research Experience Survey." *AdvanceHE*. https://s3.eu-west-2.amazonaws.com/assets.creode.advancehe-document-manager/documents/advance-he/AdvanceHE-Postgraduate_Research_%20Survey_%202019_1574338111.pdf.

Wright, R. 2008. *Native Son*. Harper Perennial Modern Classics.

Zauderer, S. 2023. "Therapist Statistics and Facts: How Many Are There?" Cross River Therapy. https://www.crossrivertherapy.com/therapist-statistics.